THINNER IN 30

THINNER IN 30

SMALL CHANGES THAT
ADD UP TO
BIG WEIGHT LOSS
IN JUST 30 DAYS

JENNA WOLFE

Lifestyle and Fitness Expert

WITH MYATT MURPHY

GRAND CENTRAL
Life & Style
NEW YORK · BOSTON

Grand Central Life & Style
Hachette Book Group
1290 Avenue of the Americas
New York, NY 10104

www.GrandCentralLifeandStyle.com

Printed in the United States of America

RRD-C

First Edition: December 2015
10 9 8 7 6 5 4 3 2 1

Grand Central Life & Style is an imprint of Grand Central Publishing.
The Grand Central Life & Style name and logo are trademarks of Hachette Book Group, Inc.

The Hachette Speakers Bureau provides a wide range of authors for speaking events. To find out more, go to www.HachetteSpeakersBureau.com or call (866) 376-6591.

The publisher is not responsible for websites (or their content) that are not owned by the publisher.

Library of Congress Cataloging-in-Publication Data

Names: Wolfe, Jenna, author.
Title: Thinner in 30 : small changes that add up to big weight loss in just
    30 days / Jenna Wolfe.
Other titles: Thinner in thirty
Description: First edition. | New York : Grand Central Life & Style, 2015. |
    Includes bibliographical references and index.
Identifiers: LCCN 2015028837| ISBN 9781455533985 (hardback) | ISBN
    9781478960652 (audio download) | ISBN 9781455533992 (ebook)
Subjects: LCSH: Reducing diets. | Weight loss. | Exercise. | Self-care,
    Health. | BISAC: HEALTH & FITNESS / Weight Loss. | HEALTH & FITNESS /
    Exercise. | HEALTH & FITNESS / Healthy Living.
Classification: LCC RM222.2 W5843 2015 | DDC 613.2/5—dc23 LC record
available at http://lccn.loc.gov/2015028837

To my best friend and soul mate Stephanie for your boundless love, patience and feedback— and for introducing me to coffee. And to our daughters Harper Estelle and Quinn Lily, the two best things that have ever happened to me. (Growing my bangs out was a close third.)

Contents

Introduction

The Start of Change

An actual conversation with my mom

MOM: Hey, Gigi! [My nickname from a million years ago when my then little brother couldn't pronounce *Jenna* so he called me *Gigi*. Yes, it sounds nothing like Jenna, but nobody ever had the heart to tell him.]

ME: Hi, Mom. What's going on?

MOM: Hey, how do I lose that extra flab under my arm when I wave? It's like I wave and then the under part of my arm waves too.

ME: Oh! I've got some great triceps exercises you can do to tighten up that area! All it takes is a few minutes a day, maybe three days a week, and I could have you try four or five different routines so you're never bored. What do you say?

(*Dead silence.*)

MOM: I think I'll just stop waving.

I'm going to be honest with you: When my agent first approached me with the idea of writing a lifestyle/fitness book, I was a little taken aback. I had written blogs, paragraphs, and various sentences in my writing past, but a book?

I mean, I had definitely *read* books before and I'm pretty sure I had *purchased* books before, but did that qualify me to go out and actually *write* one? And what would I write about? A few of the possible book topics I remember considering during that initial conversation:

- Embarrassing Things That Happen on First Dates
- Sarcastic Superheroes
- Do Vegetarians Eat Animal Crackers?
- Burpees—Not a Digestive Issue (It's an actual exercise!)
- I Know Every Episode of *The Golden Girls* (more of a fact, really, but could double as a possible book topic)

Based on that list, clearly I couldn't write a book (at least not one anyone would actually read). But then I thought about it. What do I talk about with my clients more than anything else? What is the one thing I get asked about over and over again?

How do I change from the person I am to the person I want to be?

The *x*'s and *o*'s of *change*: why it's so hard, why we generally fail before we succeed, how we approach it—and, most important, how we stick to it. If the book focused on fitness in any capacity, the answer had to be yes. (If it focused on infrastructure and economic development in sub-Saharan Africa, on the other hand, then not so much.) After all, I had dedicated my life to fitness and helping people build a path toward a healthier lifestyle:

- I was a multisport varsity athlete in high school and college, so I understand why it's important to be well conditioned all year round.
- I was a sportscaster for twelve years covering professional athletes, so I had an opportunity to see close up what the human body is capable of with the right amount of training.
- I'm a certified personal trainer, so I understand how our muscles work and how to develop individualized programs.
- I've been working with clients of all different ages, body types, and fitness levels for years, so I know what works…and what doesn't.
- I lost all my baby weight…twice…so I've been there and done that.
- And I was most recently the NBC Lifestyle and Fitness correspondent, so I know how to connect with an audience of any size.

Watching my clients' failures and successes, I definitely experience the impact of change on a daily basis, but I want to share a story with you, something I've never really admitted to myself or anyone else, much less written down, so this will be a refreshing first.

Here's my truth, and part of my inspiration for writing this book:

After I had my first daughter, Harper, I remember counting down the days until I got the green light from my OB to go back to the gym. It was six weeks. Six weeks was the magic number in my head. I knew that if I got to Week Six and everyone was healthy, I could slowly start to refocus my attention (at least a tiny tiny tiny portion of it) on getting myself back in shape. I had been breastfeeding all along, so I was still burning calories (you can burn an extra 300–500 calories a day breastfeeding), but I wanted my pre-baby body back.

So after getting my "all clear" from the doctor, I left her office and went straight to the gym. I was so pumped to start moving, jumping, squatting, lifting, pressing, biking, lunging…to do *anything*. So I walked in, threw my stuff down, and headed over to my usual spot, where I was hoping to lose myself in sweat like old times.

But that didn't happen.

The old times were clearly no longer. I couldn't start. I just stood there. Staring in the mirror. Looking at this unrecognizable body of mine.

I wasn't fat. I was…post-baby plump. But I guess I hadn't seen myself like this before…under the gym lights, without the security of my maternity clothes. I felt overwhelmed.

For the last six weeks, people had been telling me how great I looked after having the baby, and maybe I bought into it without really earning the compliment, because looking at myself in that mirror I certainly didn't feel great.

"It's such an uphill climb," I thought. "How will I ever get back to the way I used to look? And what if I can't get there? What if I lost my motivation?" Clearly all I was capable of doing that day was a slow and easy workout, but I knew that slow and easy wouldn't make me any friends. I'd have to do 5,000 mountain climbers to come even close to a decent workout (a purely irrational thought). So…what's the point?

And then it hit me.

It's not supposed to be easy. Day One of any sort of change, much less this one, is a monumental act of courage. I know it because I was there. Standing in front of a mirror, completely exposed, staring up the hill with what felt like lead legs.

All those times I had rallied my clients around the concept of "one day at a time." All those sessions when I had told them that if you change *nothing*, nothing changes. All those moments I preached that even the shortest workout on the tough days is better than nothing.

And yet there I stood…and did just that…Nothing.

Just like so many people standing at the starting gate on Day One, I was terrified to start and finally understood their fear. I finally realized that people don't refuse change because they're lazy. They refuse it because they're scared. I was afraid to fail so I was afraid to start.

Every ounce of every fiber of my being wanted to run home, put on my loose maternity clothes, and hide in my apartment. But how could I ever expect to see a change if I decided not to make one? I saw that on the back of a bus one day and never understood what it meant until that moment.

So even though I was wearing three sports bras (if you've ever tried to work out while breastfeeding, you'll know why) and a baggy T-shirt with cut-off sweats (the least motivational outfit ever). And despite being a *little* sore from having had a baby exactly six weeks prior (did you notice that *little* was in italics?), I forced myself to look at the frightened girl in the mirror. I stared at her insecurities, her postpartum frustrations, and her bigger body, and just when I thought I couldn't stand there anymore, I said out loud: "*I can and I will.*"

I can and I will.

I can and I will.

I can and I will.

I kept saying it over and over until I finally moved, until I was able to get myself down on the floor and start working out. I thought I could do 200 mountain climbers right off the bat. I did 50. And you know what? That was OK by me because at least I did something. I started and did something.

I continued to push myself for forty-five long, grueling minutes. And when I was done, I grabbed my stuff, said goodbye to the girl staring back at me in the mirror, and headed home. Day One was over. And unless I wanted another Day

One a few weeks down the road, I knew I needed to get right back to the gym to see Day Two, Day Three, Day Four, and so on.

Because I *could*—and I *would*—and I *did*.

I relied on each and every one of the thirty Changes to get back in shape after having both of my kids. I've used them with my friends, my family, and my clients to help them all lose weight and improve their health. They've worked for me, they've worked for them, and now, they're yours.

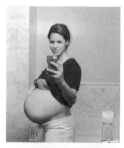

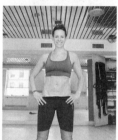

With that…a book was born. And you can thank that conversation with my mom for reminding me of my relationship with change. You see, my mom wanted to lose the flab under her arms, but she didn't want to do the work because it felt like it would be too much—and I get that.

Exercise can be intimidating.

The moves hurt.

Diets don't last.

Pizza is delicious.

I can go on and on.

We are cut from a cultural cloth where we don't start our diets 'til Monday, we vow to lose thirty pounds in a week and when the going gets tough, we just postpone getting in shape until next month or until the weather gets warmer—whichever comes second. And as a trainer, both in my personal life and on TV, I am constantly having the following conversation with people:

PERSON: How do I lose twenty pounds?

ME: Well, twenty pounds is kinda lofty. Can you start with five pounds?

PERSON: You won't notice five on me. I need to lose twenty by the summer.

ME: Riiiiight. Do you work out?

PERSON: I want to, but it's really hard because of my kids. And also, I have no time, no money, no space, no idea what to do, no desire to get up early, no good gym clothes, no trainer, no iPod, no good songs, et cetera.

ME: Et cetera? Really? OK, well how's your diet?

PERSON: I've tried Atkins, the Zone, vegan, South Beach, Jenny Craig, Mediterranean, Weight Watchers, and even bathing in lemon juice with garlic, and I just can't seem to stick to anything.

ME: (*Stunned silence*)

It takes more than just *wanting to improve* to see results. It takes energy and willpower and failure and a little sweat and a few tears, but most important, it takes time, patience, and commitment. Change doesn't happen in a day. If it did, we'd all be perfect from Day One.

But if you adjust your expectations and approach change the right way (not by swearing to lose four hundred pounds by Thursday), it's doable. And if you take the big word *change* and break it up into thirty little pieces, it suddenly becomes more manageable.

That's the approach with this book. All I'm asking you to do is make thirty small changes in your life. I won't ask you to give up everything you know on Day One and wish you the best. Instead, I've weeded through the junk out there and eliminated the impractical, separated the science, and packed each chapter with the things you need to know in the right order. Best of all, I'm even letting you decide the pace, so there's no pressure to perform and no one watching over your shoulder.

You now have an opportunity to change the one thing that everyone is dying to change, yet so few people do—their life.

You can do this.

We can do this.

Let's take this journey together, and by the time we're done, you won't need me—or anyone's help—when it comes to living a better, healthier lifestyle.

The bottom line is simple. One step at a time, one day at a time, one result at a time...OK, I'm terrible at math. But I know that it all adds up to a better you, and if I can get my parents to buy into this concept, I can get anyone to do it.

How the Change Adds Up

If I gave you thirty days' worth of diet, fitness, health, wellness, and sleep tips to chew on all at once, you'd choke, spit them out, and seek solace in your nearest waffle. Just like if I planned a month of diet and exercise goals for my mom, she'd overheat before I got to the end of the suggestion. (Still love you, Mom!)

Sure, you'd love to lose twelve pounds before your sister's wedding tomorrow. One can dream, right? And obviously you'd love to tighten up every ounce of flab by tonight (a ridiculous goal unless you went back and started the journey thirty days ago utilizing some yet-to-be-invented form of time travel, in which case reading this book would not be your biggest priority).

But what if thirty days ago was right now? What if I gave you one small way to improve an area of your life each day—every day—for thirty days? And all you would have to do is follow that lesson to the letter and carry it with you to the next day, and the next day...and so on.

Suddenly, before you knew it...*change!*

That was my motivation for the 30-Day Fitness Challenge I created for the *Today* show in 2014. We started a daily newsletter and, every day of the month, challenged viewers to make better, healthier decisions through an on-air story, a blog, or an online video with tips, tricks, and tools. The idea was that if you followed along, by the end of the month you would change your life by moving more, eating less, and making wiser decisions about your health.

One small change.

Every day.

For one month.

Within a week, I started receiving letters and e-mails from folks all over the country sharing success stories. For the first time, these viewers were feeling good about the person they saw in the mirror. It made me feel great. It made them feel great.

Now it's your turn.

I'm not asking the impossible or the improbable here. The way I see it, if you live to be eighty—about the average lifespan of an American woman—you're alive on this planet for approximately 29,200 days. Of those, I'm asking you to take just thirty and try this plan. Obviously, you'd rather do it in one day as opposed to thirty, but you and I and everyone I've ever met (and everyone you've ever met) know that's impossible.

No matter what road led you here...

- I need to lose this baby weight.
- I hate looking older than my actual age.
- I wish I had more energy to do things with my kids.
- I'd love to see my six-pack—for the first time in my life.
- I don't want to have a heart attack at forty.

...I'm just happy you're here—period. All I ask is that you be patient. Let this work for you. Let your body adjust to the little changes and give it time to do so. Don't rush something so important. For that reason, instead of telling you to change everything about your life overnight, we're going to start with one thing.

And then another.

And then another.

We'll make small, seemingly insignificant tweaks to your overall lifestyle that may not bring you results right away—but they will make a big difference as you go through the month. That's because these thirty Changes will have a cumulative effect on your life. By the end of the program, you will be leading a healthier lifestyle, feeling more fit and active, sleeping better and moving better—all without feeling like it was too much effort.

One final thing before you start: You may notice that this program isn't as precise as many you may have tried. The truth is, you don't have to overcomplicate changing your life by counting calories, carbs, grams, pounds, percentages...and other things that make your head hurt. Too often, I see experts put together complex diets and exercise programs that ask you to eat 20 percent of this type of food, or count exactly this number of calories at exactly this time of day.

Not here. Not in my book.

I promise no math, no brain bruising, and no calculations.

Good?

Let's start.

The Right Way to Count Your Change

Most diet/fitness/lifestyle books waste your time with so many studies using so many big words and so many pages before you get some information that you've lost interest before ever getting started.

My job—whether I'm working one-on-one training someone at the gym or working one-on-millions on TV—isn't explaining the whos, wheres, or whats. It's to briefly explain the whys, then get right to the hows, so that whoever I'm speaking to can get started today.

What You'll Find in Each Chapter

Simply Put...

Nothing annoys me more than when I have to read through eighteen pages of fluff just to find out the author is asking me to eat more vegetables. It's a waste of time, because all I want to know is what I need to do, so I can start doing it right away.

That's why each chapter starts with a short paragraph called Simply Put. It's basically my point for that entire chapter in a nutshell, so that you never have to comb through countless pages trying to figure out exactly what I'm asking of you.

Don't Stop There...

Some of the thirty Changes are fine on their own, while others can sometimes be taken to a whole different level—if you're up to it. Whenever that's the case, this is the section that will steer you in the right direction.

Tips and Tricks

Let's face it, we all need them. They're fun, they fit in your pocket—they're handy little life hacks that can help guide you along the often bumpy path you're about to embark on. As long as you do each little Change, you're set. But you can still use these tips and tricks to help get you there faster. So feel free to use all or some (or none) if they keep you moving forward.

The "So You Know" Science

Even though I'm a trainer, an exercise expert, and formerly the *Today* show's lifestyle and fitness correspondent, I wouldn't expect you to take my word on everything I'm advising you to change about your life. As a journalist, I know when the details can make the difference, and that's what this section is all about.

Don't worry—you won't find them in every chapter. You'll find these short but sweet nuggets of information only among Changes where knowing a little bit extra may be to your benefit. You can choose to ignore them, educate yourself by reading them, or impress your friends with your ever-growing knowledge of fitness, diet, and health.

The Only Rules to Remember

Rule #1: Once You Learn Each Change, Don't Stop Doing It as You Move Forward

All thirty Changes add up to a healthier you. Each one becomes something you'll start to do every day. Once you feel comfortable adapting to it, you can move on to the next. But to see the most results, you can't slack off. In the early chapters, the Changes can be easier to follow because you've learned only a handful. But the further you move through the book, it can sometimes be tricky to keep track, and I don't want you to let any Changes learned earlier fall to the side and be forgotten.

That's why each Change chapter starts with "Simply Put." Each day, you can quickly scroll through the book and be reminded of what you need to do, just in case that Change hasn't become second nature to you just yet.

Rule #2: Please Do Them in Order

The goal of this book—and the reason you're reading it in the first place—is to change your life. To make this plan as successful as possible for you, I put the thirty Changes in an order that works for your mind, your body, and your soul. The Changes are in an order that will not only ease you into the next Change but help you stick with all thirty long after we've finished this journey together.

Could you skip around and start with Change #3, then do Change #8, come back to Change #2, and then try Change #23? Theoretically I guess you could. But when you were young, would it have been smart to go into sixth grade before you ever went to third? Sure, you could have struggled through it, but there's a lot that you wouldn't understand or be ready for.

Going in order will also prevent you from taking any shortcuts. You could flip through this book and say to yourself, "You know what? This Change works with my schedule, but this Change doesn't right now, so I'll come back to it." But you probably won't.

Doing them out of sequence, or picking and choosing what works best for you and ignoring what doesn't, will only put you at risk of failing, because there's a lot your mind and body may not be ready for. It also makes it easier to ignore certain key Changes that will most likely have the greatest impact on your life.

Rule #3: Move at Your Own Pace

Thirty days is the least amount of time it should take to get through all of the Changes—adopting one new Change each day for thirty days. Some will be easier (enjoy those and don't skip over them because you already "know that one").

Life isn't a dress rehearsal and it's certainly not a race. You don't have to rush through this. If you kept failing at various diet/fitness plans, think about why that was. Were you trying to do too much too soon too drastically? Make this work so that never happens again. Take your time and do this right and watch yourself stick to it for a change.

So you can do all of this in thirty days. Or, if you want to make a Change every other day, every four days, every week, or every other week, I won't stop you from setting your own pace. If it takes you a little more time to adapt to a Change, by all means spend time on it. And if you have to go backward because a Change didn't quite stick, then I want you to go back without feeling bad about it.

This book is merely a guide, a guide I've put together that takes you from what is simplest to incorporate into your life to what is slightly more complicated. I used this plan to lose all my baby weight. I know it works. I've seen it work.

Count the Changes—Not the Pounds

In this book, you'll find many numbers, ranging from how many sips of water I expect you to drink each morning to how many things you should check off your "I WILL DO" list each day. But there's one number I don't want you to be defined by, and that's your weight.

You won't find one piece of advice in this book that asks you to use your bodyweight as a barometer. Why? Because so many people become so fixated on weight that they can never pay attention to the positive things that are happening to them and around them.

They never notice that their pants suddenly fit better or that they can perform a squat effortlessly. They never realize that they're now able to walk five miles a day or that they have stopped succumbing to their sugar cravings. In other words, they never notice the countless changes happening to them because they stay fixated on the only thing they want to change—that number on the scale.

I'm not saying that you can't weigh yourself, but there are so many other barometers besides the scale. Through this book, you are going to reteach your body how to live, eat, sleep, and function—and it's a process that takes time. So don't let that number between your feet when you step onto the scale define you. Instead, define yourself by how many Changes you have under your belt.

#1

Drink 20 Sips of Water the Moment You Wake Up

SIMPLY PUT . . . Put a full glass of water by your bed before you go to sleep each night. When your alarm goes off in the morning, literally sit up and start drinking. Drink twenty normal-sized sips of water. Not after breakfast or with your coffee. Not over the course of the morning, or on the way to work, or sometime throughout the day. Not in the shower or the— Please don't drink your shower water as your morning beverage. The alarm goes off, you sit up, reach for that glass, and drink.

Seems almost too easy, doesn't it? But the few seconds you'll spend sitting there on the edge of your bed sipping away will actually do your body hours of good afterward.

What you're doing by taking those twenty sips is more than most people ever bother doing. You're waking up your metabolism and literally telling your body "OK, here's the deal: It's time to get moving because we've got a lot of work to do today. I need you to start revving up so that anything I eat is digested properly and I'm burning as many calories as possible when I finally get out of this bed." I know that sounds like a lot to tell yourself, but you've been quiet all night: It's time to unleash the Chatty Cathy in you.

You see, every time you wake up, your body is already starting the day at a disadvantage by being dehydrated. Don't worry—it's a natural thing from not having anything to drink for six to eight hours (made even worse if you're the type that wakes up a lot at night to pee).

The problem is, most people do nothing about it, and losing as little as 1 percent of your bodyweight in water not only slows down your body's metabolism, it also causes fatigue that prevents you from being as active as you could be. Being dehydrated may even be behind your bad early-morning eating habits, especially if you're the type that eats everything in sight as soon as the sun's up. That's because when you're parched, your body oftentimes mistakes that thirst for hunger. Your body's not as smart as you are. (No offense, body.)

Taking those twenty sips will kick-start your metabolism and even curb some of your hunger pangs, so you're burning calories from the get-go. Right off the bat, those twenty sips give you a little bit of time to ease into the morning. Your body is a machine and you just fueled it, not with food but just by doing something so few people ever consider—you're hydrating it.

My favorite reason behind those twenty sips is how they set the table for many of the other changes in this book. They force you to do something good for yourself before you even think about what you need to handle for your family, your boss, or whoever else wants a piece of you that day. They will remind you of what's ahead and give you time to reflect and prepare for the other changes you'll soon learn and incorporate into your lifestyle.

DON'T STOP THERE...

So why twenty?

If you need a study where researchers in Tajikistan discovered that drinking exactly twenty sips was the ideal number to consume, I really have nothing for you. The truth is, twenty is just the number of sips I've found most people can commit to, and it's an easy way to get people to start drinking water right away.

Once you're committed—and you begin to feel the positive effects of rehydrating yourself every morning—you won't want to lose that feeling. You'll begin to find yourself going "beyond the twenty sips" and hydrating consistently from morning until night (whether you're thirsty or not). Which is a good thing, because staying hydrated will crush your crazy cravings, leave you feeling fuller longer, and reduce your appetite for excess calories during every meal. It will also help your body figure out whether it's really hungry or just really bored.

I promise you that after a couple of days or weeks, you'll start to see that you're not as hungry as you thought you were. Sometimes you're simply eating out of sheer boredom, nervousness, or depression. Most of all, you'll find yourself surprised to learn how much water your body truly needs over the course of the day, and how little you're actually giving it.

Ideally, I'd like to have you drink a minimum of half of your bodyweight (in ounces) in water throughout the day. For example, if you weigh 160 pounds, that would be 80 ounces a day (160/2 is 80). I believe the problem is that most people tend to get hung up on how many bottles, glasses, and ounces they need to drink each day. That's way too much thinking. If I asked you to drink eight glasses of water a day, at eight ounces of water a glass, you'd have to tap into math, and nobody should have to do that *and* try to eat healthy at the same time, right?

So for now, just follow some of the simple tricks in this chapter. And I promise you, you'll reach that "half your bodyweight" goal unconsciously and automatically without ever needing to break out a calculator, abacus, checklist, or app.

Tips and Tricks

No counting glasses or breaking out measuring cups. All I want you to do is give a few of these habit-forming recommendations a try:

Find the biggest beaker you can bear. Don't settle for whatever-sized glasses are in your cabinets. Sure, I could drink 280 cups of water from my kid's little sippy cup. It's the size of a thimble!! Either buy one that's much larger or make a habit of drinking from a liter-sized bottle of water. If you sit behind a desk, make sure you keep a large bottle right in front of you. If you're driving most of the day, keep it in your car. Challenge yourself to refill it a certain number of times each day depending on its size. See how many days in a row you can keep up with that number. Each time you empty it, you'll have thrown back more than you might have otherwise.

Never leave your glass empty. Make a habit of stopping to refill whatever you're drinking from the moment you finish it—no excuses—even if you're not planning on drinking any more after that. Just having a full container with you will increase your odds of drinking more later.

Fill it and chill it. Grab a pitcher, pour the amount of water I want you to eventually drink each day (half your bodyweight in ounces), and just leave it in the fridge. Just seeing it may inspire you to compete against yourself to see if you can finish it by day's end.

Put time on your side. Every time you check to see what time it is, sneak in a sip of water. In my mom's case, every time she checks the weather, I have her drinking water. She's now officially part fish. And she's obsessed with the weather for some reason.

Put a bottle in several places. If you find yourself in different spots during the day, even in your own house, don't settle for drinking from one bottle or glass. Instead, put one in several areas. That way, if you forget to bring your water with you, you'll always have some handy.

Sip during your guilty pleasures. Choose an activity (or several) that you either tend to do frequently or love to do, like checking social media, reading your e-mails, or watching your favorite TV shows. I won't judge how you're passing your time, so long as you sip.

Tack a 5 or 10 onto that 20. Adding a few extra sips onto your morning ritual will only reenergize your body even more, speed up digestion, and let you reach your daily quota of water even faster.

Have it on ice for extra results. Your body has to heat up every sip to match your constant temperature of around 98.6 degrees. Experts say that the extra effort can burn between 1 and 8 calories per 8 ounces.

Use a straw. As strange as it sounds, people tend to mindlessly drink more and take much larger gulps when sipping through one. Try one of those crazy curly oversized straws; they're fun, except during big important unplanned meetings with your boss and your boss's boss. I learned that lesson the hard way...but I got my sips in!

Try it fizzy. Seltzer water still counts, so if having a bit of fizz makes you more likely to sneak in sips all day, bring it on.

Add some heat to what you eat. Splashing a little hot sauce or adding some crushed red pepper to certain foods isn't just a commonsense trick to get you drinking more: Hot peppers also give your metabolism a natural boost.

Finally, dress it up! Water can be boring—I get that. So make it more interesting by adding some flavor to it. But don't use those man-made flavoring products that you squirt into a glass. You can try freezing small chunks of peeled oranges, lemons, or limes and using them instead of an ice cube, or mix in a hint of vanilla extract to make drinking water more enticing.

Better yet, it takes almost zero effort to make your own "spa-inspired" water by infusing a pitcher of water with chunks of fruit, veggies, spices, and herbs. Infuse-friendly ingredients that work include

- Fruit: Apples, berries (any kind, either fresh or frozen), cherries, citrus and/ or tropical fruits (grapefruit, kiwis, lemons, limes, oranges, and pineapples, for example), melon (any kind), and pears
- Herbs and edible flowers: Basil leaves, cilantro leaves, lavender, lemongrass, mint leaves, parsley, rose petals, rosemary sprigs, sage, and thyme. Avoid using all at one time (I learned that lesson the hard way).
- Spices: Cardamom pods, cinnamon sticks, cloves, fennel bulb (sliced), ginger (sliced), and vanilla bean (seedless)
- Vegetables: Carrots, celery, cucumber, and yes, even jalapeño peppers

If that list sounds daunting, relax. It's practically dummy proof to drink like a diva. Just grab a pitcher (jars and large glass bottles with lids are great too) and toss in thinly sliced pieces or small cubes of whatever combination of things you want to try. Just be sure it's fresh and not ripe or bruised. Fill the container close to the top with ice and cold water (filtered is always best), throw it in the fridge, let it sit a few hours (the longer, the better—although twenty-four hours really starts to push it), and that's honestly it.

Need a few combination suggestions? No matter what your tastes, you're sure to find something here that will keep you unconsciously reaching more often for more aqua:

- Cider: Mix several cored, thinly sliced apples with several whole cinnamon sticks.
- Cucumber-Lime: Mix 1 small cucumber (thinly sliced), ½ a sliced lime, and toss in a few mint leaves.
- Orange-Blueberry: Mix 2 oranges (cut in 8 wedges) and a handful of blueberries.
- Pear Surprise: Mix several cored, thinly sliced pears and either 8 to 12 pieces of thinly sliced fresh ginger or a thinly sliced fennel bulb.
- Strawberry-Lemon: Mix 4 to 5 strawberries (take the tops off, then quarter them), ½ a lemon (thinly sliced), and a few leaves of basil (bruising them first will bring out their flavor).

The "So You Know" Science

Staying hydrated from Minute One of your morning does a lot more than just jump-start your metabolism and keep cravings at bay.

Waiting until you're thirsty before you drink means your body has probably already lost 4 to 5 percent of its total water. That's why you can't rely on being thirsty as a gauge. By the time you're thirsty, you're already dehydrated to some extent. And that's no place to find yourself, since every function within your body requires water to some extent. Staying topped off keeps everything running at full speed, so that every single function taking place throughout your body—from digestion and circulation to regulating your blood pressure and body temperature—runs smoothly.

Water is also your best workout partner, especially if your goal is to lose weight. Beyond keeping you from overheating during intense exercise, having your tank filled helps your body process protein (making it easier to build and maintain lean muscle), transport nutrients and oxygen to your cells, and flush away toxins and waste left behind when your body breaks down fat for energy.

But skip the sips and all that support gets downgraded. Even worse, one classic study published in the *Journal of Strength and Conditioning Research* found that a loss in water of as little as 2 percent of your bodyweight can significantly affect both your strength and endurance. That's not a good thing, especially since you'll need both for the workouts in this book later on. Making a habit of being well hydrated now will mean you'll have more energy to put into the exercise programs to come—and you can expect to see better results for all your hard work.

Today show Tested

As one of my *Today* show assignments, I was given the task of converting my former colleague, national investigative correspondent Jeff Rossen, from a diet soda aficionado to a water-drinking machine. To say I had my work cut out for me was an understatement, as Rossen lived on diet soda. So I started him off with twenty sips of water every morning, and as you might imagine, I was met with the following text every eight minutes: "Going to the bathroom...AGAIN!!"

After a week, the texts subsided (thankfully) and the water intake grew from twenty morning sips to a few bottles a day to water all day long. Rossen saw firsthand that filling up on water before a meal, before a big night out, before a tempting plate of food, cut his appetite and thus cut calories. (He could also tell you the exact location of every bathroom at the *Today* show studios with his eyes closed.) This simple Change, in combination with a few others we'll get to in the next few chapters, helped him lose almost fifteen pounds in a month.

#2
Start a Food Diary

SIMPLY PUT...I want you to write down everything you eat. Not "some" things. Not "most" things. *Everything*—every last morsel of food and beverage you put into your mouth from the time you wake up until the time you go to bed. It doesn't matter if it's a bite of toast, two sips of a latte, or five M&Ms, write it all down. (You'll quickly realize it's easier to just skip the M&Ms than to write down that you ate five...*FIVE*???) Don't count calories. Don't bother tracking how many grams of protein, carbs, or fats are tucked inside whatever you're eating. Just write down everything you've consumed. At the end of the day, e-mail it to a friend (or a group of friends...or your enemies...or your friends' enemies) willing to do the same.

An actual conversation with my mom

ME: Hey, Mom, how's your food diary coming along?

MOM: It's good. I wrote down what I ate for lunch yesterday and I guess I didn't need the two cookies I had afterwards.

ME: See? That's how it works! You hold yourself accountable and you—

MOM: And those Wise potato chips.

ME: OK, well yeah, those aren't great. But again, that's how it works. When you write—

MOM: Your father had a slice of frozen cheesecake for dessert.

The only way any of this is going to work—the only way every Change in this book will eventually become a part of your lifestyle—is if you hold yourself accountable. And the best way to do that is by literally watching, and eventually controlling, what you eat.

Let's face it: If you never answer for the things you do, it's easy to cheat, skip steps, avoid what you hate doing, and do whatever you want, whenever you want. What you're left with is square one, and haven't we all ended up there far too often? In order to curb what you're eating, you have to first *know* what you're eating. And in order to know what you're eating, you have to log it.

Plain and simply, this is how I lost the bulk of my weight after I had my first baby. No crazy diets or crash cleanses or five-hour workout sessions. I started a food diary and every night, I e-mailed it to my three best buds at the *Today* show (Lester Holt, Erica Hill, and Dylan Dreyer). They in turn sent me theirs, and what ensued was a three-month stretch of self-monitoring everything we ate and making appropriate healthy changes.

We all lost weight, despite a somewhat stubborn start by our dear pal Lester, who held on tight to his favorite dessert of crème brûlée until he surrendered to the power of the diary a week in and switched over to fruit. That's when he was hooked. My aha moment came by Week Three, when I was eating salads for breakfast as a chest-pounding, competitively strategic move. It didn't exactly catch on, but for that special week my fiber intake was through the roof.

Keeping a food diary is the ultimate accountable step. Quite honestly, monitoring what goes into your body is one of the single most important things you can do for yourself, one that asks so little effort in return. And before you complain that it's no fun jotting every single thing down, ask yourself this: Is it any less fun than trying to squeeze into the jeans that no longer fit you or the sweater you used to live in because it was so loose and cozy? (BTW, my post-baby body tried on that same sweater and wondered when it had turned into spandex.) Within two weeks of keeping a food log after my first baby, I not only got into a food-logging groove, I was starting to make wiser food choices without so much as a word of guidance from anyone or having to make a conscious effort to do so.

DON'T STOP THERE...

Look, I'm not asking you to draw a diagram, add up calories, or scribble down any of the information from the back label of whatever you've inhaled. What you choose to eat and drink isn't important. To be truthful, none of that matters to me right now. This is just about writing down everything you're eating and drinking all day long. That's all. The change—your adjustment—will come on its own.

Just write down every little speck of food and drink from sunup until bedtime. I don't care if it's the three raisins you picked off your kid's plate. I don't care if it's half a bite of half a pizza crust. All I can say is: If you found the need to put that half a bite in your mouth, then you need to write it down and hold yourself accountable for it.

Now, you can use what I'm asking of you in a couple of different ways. You can jot down everything you eat and drink, stare at the list at the end of the day, and sit with the choices you've made on your own. That's not a bad plan. In fact, research has shown that dieters who keep a food diary tend to do better when it comes to meeting and beating their weight-loss goals compared to those who can't be bothered.

But what I like to do is bring others onboard for the ride.

Everyone has friends in the same boat. They either need to lose weight, want to get healthy, or sit somewhere in between. (I should really be calling it a cruise ship, given the number of friends aboard who want to join in on my next food diary.) And when you're sharing that list with a group or even on social media, you'll start making smarter choices a lot faster without trying that hard. It all comes down to the fact that when you know other people will be looking at what and how you're eating, you'll be less inclined to fill your list with junk.

It also brings out your competitive spirit, no matter who you are. You may not care who's eating what in the beginning. But mark my words: If one friend sends back a food diary with a huge salad on it, and you're staring down an endless bowl of mac 'n' cheese, I can guarantee you won't be dining with Ms. Mary Mac (and cheese) tonight.

As the days go by, you'll slowly start making wiser choices, cleaner choices, and better choices. You'll automatically start making dietary decisions based on what other people are reading about you and what they're sending you. After all, nobody wants to be the loser in the group who caved and had two Pop-Tarts at three in the afternoon (even if they're Frosted Strawberry).

That said, the rules are painless enough:

1. Find someone who (or a group of people that) will do this with you for the long haul, not anyone that could really care less and may be doing it just to help you out. Preferably, find people with the same goals as you (to become healthier, to get in great shape, and if needed, lose a little weight).
2. Be honest. If you cheat, I swear you're only cheating yourself. Those jeans will never fit you unless you actually *eat* the salads and don't just *lie* about eating the salads.
3. Finally, be consistent. That means starting on the exact same day and e-mailing your friend or friends as soon as you finish your last bite for the night, no matter if it's six p.m. or midnight—you'll find yourself wanting to finish first just to beat out your friend who somehow finds a way every night to get her diary in by six p.m. even though she has two hungry kids and a husband and an amazing pantry of snacks and…Sorry, I digress.

Tips and Tricks

You'll be amazed how something as simple and effortless as seeing words on a page will affect you. But if you need help staying the course—or want to turn your food diary into something even more meaningful—here are just a few easy ways to do exactly that.

Snap a pic and send it. In addition to writing down every detail, grab your phone, then take a picture of your meals and snacks and immediately send it to your friends. Revealing what you're eating in the moment (and seeing what they're eating as well) may fire up your competitive spirit even more.

Choose what works best for you. Don't feel like lugging around a journal? Then text yourself. Can't type 911 without misspelling it? Then carry scrap paper in your pocket. The point: just use whatever's easiest for you. I don't care if it's a Post-it note or the back of your hand—just so long as you write down every crumb, you're fine.

Give yourself a break one week a month. If you want to see how powerful a tool a food diary is, write everything down for three weeks, then take one week off. You'll immediately notice that during your time off, you'll end up eating and drinking so much more compared to the weeks prior that you'll eventually want to track what you ingest all the time.

Don't be selective about your days. If you have some big occasion where eating mass quantities of food is unfortunately unavoidable, that's no time to take off. These are the crucial days when holding yourself liable matters most—so double down.

Write down what you eat before you eat it. Seeing certain foods in print before you pound them back may help you eat less of the bad stuff and more of the good. Why? It gives you time to reflect and ask yourself, "Do I really want to commit to this? Am I proud of what's on this paper?" When the answer's no, you may find yourself dialing back on what makes you feel guilty.

Don't be afraid to fire your friends. If you ever start to feel like your diary buddies are cutting you way too much slack, or they've lost their motivation to stick things out, confide in someone new.

Blame it on your health. If you're too self-conscious about what others may think and don't want to come off seeming weight-obsessed, tell them you're doing this to get healthy. You'll be surprised how fast the gossip stops when people think you're watching what you eat to lower your cholesterol or have more energy to play with your kids.

Don't ignore the extras. Coming clean with every scrap of food also means being accountable for whatever you've smeared, squirted, or shaken on top of it. So don't ignore recording any sauces, spreads, condiments, sugar, or sugar substitutes—even if you don't think it has a single calorie in it, own up to it.

If you can handle the details, then do it. Writing down the names of what you're eating is all I expect from you. But for some, going beyond the bare minimum can help explore triggers that could be behind some of your food choices and habits. Just a few things you may want to track before and after every meal could include

- Your energy levels
- Your mood
- The time of day (and how much time you've waited between meals)
- Your location
- Your level of hunger

#3

Walk 10,000 Steps a Day

SIMPLY PUT . . . Strap on an activity bracelet or an inexpensive pedometer and track how many steps you actually take in a day. Whatever that number is, add to it until you get to at least 10,000.

Here's why: Since walking burns around 100 calories/mile and a mile is around 2,000 steps, walking 10,000 steps a day equals 5 miles and burns close to 500 calories (extra if you weigh more than average). That equals 3,500 calories a week (or one pound) and 182,000 calories a year!!!

If 10,000 steps a day sounds like a lot, first consider that the average person is already walking roughly more than 5,000 steps daily. So you're already more than halfway there. Then consider that there is no easier exercise assignment than "walk more," so appreciate it now while we're in the early Changes.

And if 10,000 steps a day happens to be a few extra outside your comfort zone, fantastic. I love that space. That's where all the good stuff happens. That's where you take chances and face your fears and that's where real change occurs. While the rest of the world relies on the safety and warmth of their comfort zone, I want you to spend a little time each day outside it.

Forcing yourself to reach 10k steps is one way to do that.

To track all those steps, you don't have to go out and buy a multifunctional exercise fitness bracelet or watch, especially if you don't have the money or don't need any of the other technologies typically built into them. Instead, just go to the drugstore and buy yourself a ten-dollar pedometer.

Yeah, it may not look as fashionable (my mom wears one that could easily double as a wall clock, but she gets her steps in!) and it may not be 100 percent accurate, but even those high-tech fitness trackers aren't all calibrated in exactly the same way. If you wore five on each arm and walked a mile, I'll guarantee none of them would come up with the exact same number of steps. Even if your pedometer is off by 1,000 footsteps, it's fine. You won't be doing any athletic disservice to yourself. Remember, you're only using it as a gauge.

Once you have something to track your steps, start moving and figure out how much walking you need to do to reach 10k. At the end of the day, if you only see the number 8,000 sadly blinking back at you, well...I'm sorry to tell you this but you're 2,000 steps shy. (No, Mom, you can't "make it up tomorrow.") Find a way to reach your goal before you go to bed.

Get moving and reach that 10,000-step finish line before the end of the day, whether it takes walking around your house, hiking up and down your staircase, or marching in place during commercial breaks. ("No fast-forwarding through commercials!!" said literally nobody, except the person aiming for 10,000 steps.) And trust me, the first time that happens to you, the first time you're saddled with cramming in last-minute steps just to hit 10k, your walking habits will change almost immediately. The next day, you'll actively look for ways to get those missed 2,000 steps in a lot earlier.

Ways to Get Your Steps in...

- Choose a subway/bus/train stop or parking spot farther from your office.
- Use a bathroom on a different floor at work.
- Walk around the practice field watching your kids play sports instead of just bench warming.
- Pace while you're on the phone.
- Find the farthest parking space at a store—the one no one uses unless it's Black Friday and the lot's full.
- Never use another drive-thru again. It's either walk in or you get nothing.

- Anytime you're forced to stand or sit and wait for anything, opt to walk or march in place instead. You'll get steps in and you'll look cool. Well…Let's just say you'll get some steps in.
- Make it a ritual to take a five-minute walk after every meal.
- Make it a habit to walk the mall three times before hitting the stores.

Two More Things to Remember…

In addition to my 10k steps, there are two things I do all the time that have made a huge difference in my life, two things that used to be a challenge for me but now just come naturally.

- One is <u>keeping my stomach engaged</u> throughout the day, holding it tight as if someone were about to punch me in the gut. (I'll explain this further in another Change.)
- The other is <u>contracting my gluteal muscles</u>. (Yes, that's my way of saying I'm constantly squeezing my butt cheeks whenever I walk. Clearly I'm very fancy.) It's a simple trick that secretly works the muscles that make up your derriere, and now you have 10,000 mini opportunities to do just that.

When I first tried it, I had to remind myself every few seconds, which turned into every few minutes and eventually once or twice daily. Now it's so second nature to me that even if I just get up in the middle of the night to use the bathroom, I still squeeze my glutes with every step. (An interesting visual, now that I think about it.)

It takes time and practice to get to where it will become routine for you too, but it will. And I'll be straight with you: Doing it for a few minutes a day really doesn't add up to a whole heck of a lot. But use this tactic with your 10,000 steps and you'll burn even more calories each day while simultaneously strengthening and shaping your glutes.

Tips and Tricks

Walking burns calories while strengthening your heart, legs, butt, lower back, and abdominals. Plus, it's free, safe, and one of the most joint-friendly, risk-free forms of cardiovascular activity out there. But that doesn't mean you can't eke a little more from all 10,000 steps...

Give your walks a soundtrack... In a classic study out of Ohio State University, people who listened to music while walking felt less exhausted and went about 21 percent farther than usual.

...But pick the best type of tunes. Choosing songs with a faster tempo has been shown to boost a walker's pace, so take advantage of it. (Not that I don't love Barbra Streisand, but power walking all around town to "Memories" just doesn't paint the most athletic picture.)

Quick Tip: Tap your foot with each song, then count how many times you tap your foot in one minute. For slow to moderate walks, choose songs that range between 90 and 125 beats per minute. If you're a fast walker (and want to get more steps in), stick with songs that range between 130 and 160 beats per minute.

Then arrange your songs in the right order. Don't just hit shuffle on your music player. Instead, make a playlist of your all-time favorite songs, then arrange them from least favorite to "can't live without," so your best songs won't play until about halfway through your walk. That way, you'll get a boost just when you need it most.

Don't try to lengthen your stride. Just let your feet fall where they may. Trying to take longer steps so you'll travel farther will only throw off your natural rhythm and body mechanics. To utilize all the muscles within your butt, thighs, and waist, your hips should feel as if they are rolling back and forth with your legs.

Stand straight and look forward as often as possible. Rounding your shoulders, tilting your head down, or leaning back prevents your weight from being evenly distributed, which affects how much oxygen you take in and compromises the muscles of the lower back. Instead, keep your chin lifted, back straight, and abs tight.

Give yourself a raise on the treadmill. Walk normally and your body is the only thing moving yourself forward. But on a treadmill, a motor pulls the surface backward, so your body never has to work quite as hard. Raise the incline to 1 percent so your muscles work as hard as if they were walking on a flat surface outside.

Keep an eye on your arms... Swinging your arms back and forth uses additional calories and helps counterbalance your legs to stabilize your body. Somewhere between nothing at all and the ridiculously hilarious but adorable sweeping arm swings my mom and her friends use is where I want you to live. Ideally, your elbows should be bent at a 90-degree angle. As you walk, pump your arms back and forth in a straight line (not at an angle), swinging your fists no farther forward than chest-high. As you draw them back, your fists should line up by your hips.

…Then use your arms to speed things along. Your arms act as gearshifts. The quicker you swing them back and forth, the more your pace picks up. So if you feel your feet beginning to drag, try swinging your arms faster and your legs should fall in line.

Glance down at your legs and feet. With each step, your toes, foot, ankle, knee, and hip should all be pointing straight ahead and be in line with one another. Land on the heel of each foot, roll forward onto the ball of the foot, and then push off with your toes.

If your toes seem to roll inward or outward, you could be either a pronator or supinator and may require special footwear to avoid aches and pains after this Change becomes a habit. In that case, contact a podiatrist or visit a technical shoe store that caters to runners and walkers.

Make adjustments when it's hot. High temperatures, humidity, and direct sun cause your body to overwork itself in order to keep cool. Stay safe when walking in the sun:

- Don't overexert yourself between 10:00 a.m. and 4:00 p.m. (That's when the sun is at its peak and ozone and UV rays are at their highest levels for the day.)
- Wear lighter-colored, looser-fitting clothes made from breathable materials (such as CoolMax, SmartWool, and spun polyester) and avoid darker, tight-fitting clothing made from fabrics that trap heat and moisture (like cotton).
- Always wear sunscreen, even when it's cloudy. And if you really work up a sweat on your walks, use an oil-based sunscreen instead of a water-based version so it stays on you.

The "So You Know" Science

If you think walking's weak because it's a low-intensity, low-aerobic activity, think again. Walking targets the same muscles that running does (the hamstrings, quadriceps, glutes, calves, and even the abdominals and lower back to a certain extent). And performed at an incline—either on a treadmill or up hills—walking can even burn as many calories and condition your cardiovascular system as effectively as running can, minus all the stress on your joints.

Countless studies have proven that, in addition to all the calories you'll burn, walking every day also improves your body's ability to consume oxygen, lowers blood pressure and low-density lipoprotein (LDL) cholesterol (the "bad" kind), raises high-density lipoprotein (HDL) cholesterol (the "good" kind), and it even boosts your psychological and physical well-being.

Stop Eating Simple Carbs After 6:00 p.m.

SIMPLY PUT . . . Stop eating foods rich in simple carbs at 6:00 p.m. That doesn't mean limit yourself to eating less simple carbs—I mean stop eating simple carbs altogether.

Carbs are considered good or bad depending on what kind they are and what your body does with them. There are two types of carbohydrates: simple carbs and complex carbs.

Simple carbs absorb into the blood quickly, provide a source of quick energy, and are very high in sugar. They are basically calories with few nutrients that add little real value to your body other than quick energy, and even that doesn't last very long. Some examples: bread, pasta, and sugary foods.

Complex carbs are harder for the body to break down. They are still considered carbs, but instead of the quick "sugar high" you get from simple carbs, complex carbs contain lower amounts of sugars that are released at a more consistent rate. They are typically packed with fiber, leaving you feeling fuller for a longer period of time. Some examples: whole-grain breads, starchy vegetables, and beans.

I have no problem with you eating good complex carbs after 6:00 p.m. Vegetables are some of my best friends. Also, I would never tell you to cut out an entire food group—ever. It's unrealistic, it doesn't last, I don't think it's healthy, and I'm not that cold-blooded. So when I tell you to eliminate carbs from your diet starting at 6:00 p.m., it's not because I'm steering you toward a low-carb diet or somehow I think carbs are evil.

Carbs can't tell time, and the myth that you'll gain weight because you ate carbs when the sun was down is exactly that. But when it comes to weight loss, it's all about energy eaten versus energy spent. And it's at night that we tend to do the bulk of our poor eating.

Think about it. We're so much better at controlling what we eat during the day because we have more energy and we have people around us for accountability. But after a long day of work, stress, kids, diets, decisions, directions, comings, and goings, we tend to let ourselves go—and it becomes a free-for-all.

Simple carbs are quickly absorbed by your body and packed with excess calories and sugar. So if you cap your bad carbs around dinnertime, it keeps you in check. By setting that limit, you're instantly reminding yourself to eat better, because it leaves you with no choice but to make healthier choices.

DON'T STOP THERE . . .

If six o'clock isn't challenging enough for you, then move the time up to 5:00 p.m. When that becomes doable—and it could take anywhere from a matter of days to weeks or months—then bump it up to 4:00 p.m. Whatever that comfort zone is for you, where you can realistically do this on a daily basis, I want you to play in that space.

Obviously, if you work the night shift or work odd hours, you'll have to change the rules. Instead of sticking to six o'clock, just stop eating carbs between four and five hours before you typically fall asleep.

That said, am I saying "Don't eat"? Nope. Instead, get yourself a lean piece of protein (beef, pork, fish, or poultry) and load up with as many vegetables and healthy fats as you like. Most vegetables are low-glycemic foods that are low in calories, slower to digest, and won't elevate your blood sugar—so nosh away.

The healthier carbs found in whole-grain foods, beans and grains (including quinoa, oats, whole-wheat bread, and brown rice), low-carb fruits, nuts, and seeds take a lot longer for your body to break down, plus they contain plenty of fiber.

I just don't want you even thinking about reaching for processed and/or starchy food like bread, white rice, white baked potatoes, or pasta.

I can't be there to hold your hand on this one, so let your conscience be your guide. If you're walking away from the dinner table feeling gross and ashamed about what you ate, there's probably a reason. But there's that other feeling you get when you wake up feeling proud of the way you ate—so proud that you want to do it again. And that's the feeling I want you to strive toward.

Still, if you don't trust your conscience, here are a few foods you can trust to make the change a little bit easier:

MEATS AND POULTRY		
Food	*Portion Size*	*Carbs (in grams)*
Bacon (regular)	One slice	0
Beef tenderloin (lean, boneless; roasted)	3 oz.	0
Bison (roasted)	3 oz.	0
Bottom round (lean; cooked)	3 oz.	0
Brisket (lean; braised)	3 oz.	0
Canadian bacon	3 oz.	0
Chicken breast (boneless)	3 oz.	0
Chicken breast (with bone)	3 oz.	0
Chicken thigh (boneless)	3 oz.	0
Chicken thigh (with bone)	3 oz.	0
Chuck roast (lean; braised)	3 oz.	0
Duck breast (broiled)	3 oz.	0
Eye round (lean; roasted)	3 oz.	0
Filet mignon (lean; broiled)	3 oz.	0
Flank steak (lean; braised)	3 oz.	0
Flank steak (lean; broiled)	3 oz.	0
Ground beef (70% lean/30% fat)	3 oz.	0
Ground beef (80% lean/20% fat)	3 oz.	0
Ground beef (extra lean)	3 oz.	0
Jerky (beef)	1 oz.	3
Jerky (turkey)	1 oz.	3
Lamb chop (lean; broiled)	3 oz.	0
Ostrich (ground)	3 oz.	0

MEATS AND POULTRY *(continued)*		
Food	*Portion Size*	*Carbs (in grams)*
Pheasant (whole)	3 oz.	0
Pork tenderloin (roasted)	3 oz.	0
Rib steak (lean; broiled)	3 oz.	0
Roast beef (lunch meat)	3 oz.	3
T-bone (lean; broiled)	3 oz.	0
Top round steak (braised)	3 oz.	0
Top sirloin steak (broiled)	3 oz.	0
Turkey breast (with skin; roasted)	3 oz.	0
Turkey dark meat (with skin; roasted)	3 oz.	0
Turkey leg	3 oz.	0
Veal chop (lean; braised)	3 oz.	0
Venison	3 oz.	0

SEAFOOD		
Food	*Portion Size*	*Carbs (in grams)*
Atlantic cod (baked)	3 oz.	0
Brown trout (baked)	3 oz.	0
Carp (baked)	3 oz.	0
Catfish (steamed)	3 oz.	0
Flounder (baked)	3 oz.	0
Grouper (baked)	3 oz.	0
Haddock (baked or steamed)	3 oz.	0

SEAFOOD *(continued)*

Food	Portion Size	Carbs (in grams)
Halibut (baked)	3 oz.	0
Mahimahi (baked)	3 oz.	0
Orange roughy (baked)	3 oz.	0
Salmon (baked or broiled)	3 oz.	0
Sea bass (baked)	3 oz.	0
Shrimp	3 oz.	0
Sole (baked)	3 oz.	0
Striped bass (baked)	3 oz.	0
Trout (baked)	3 oz.	0
Tuna (bluefin; baked)	3 oz.	0
Tuna (canned in water)	3 oz.	0

NUTS, SEEDS, AND DAIRY

Food	Portion Size	Carbs (in grams)
Almonds	1 oz.	6
Brazil nuts	1 oz.	3.5
Cheese (Cheddar, provolone, or Swiss)	One slice	0.5
Cottage cheese (nonfat)	4 oz.	7
Egg (whole)	One large	0
Egg (white)	One large	0
Macadamia nuts	1 oz.	4
Peanuts	1 oz.	4.5
Pecans	1 oz.	4
Pumpkin seeds (raw)	1 Tbsp.	1
Sunflower seeds	1 oz.	5
Walnuts	1 oz.	4

VEGETABLES

Food	Portion Size	Carbs (in grams)
Asparagus	4 oz.	5
Beets (cooked)	½ cup	8
Bell peppers	½ cup	5
Broccoli (steamed)	½ cup	4
Cabbage (chopped)	½ cup	3
Carrot	One (medium sized)	3

VEGETABLES *(continued)*

Food	Portion Size	Carbs (in grams)
Cauliflower	½ cup	3
Celery	½ cup	2
Corn (sweet white)	½ cup	8
Cucumber	One (8-inch)	11
Green beans	½ cup	4
Kale	½ cup	4
Lettuce (Boston, iceberg, or romaine)	Four leaves	2
Peas	½ cup	10
Portobello mushroom	One (medium sized)	0.5
Snow peas (steamed)	½ cup	6
Spinach (cooked)	½ cup	3.5
Tomato	One (medium sized)	7
Zucchini (steamed)	½ cup	3

FRUITS

Food	Portion Size	Carbs (in grams)
Apricot (fresh or dried)	One	4
Avocado	¼ cup	3
Blackberries	½ cup	7
Cantaloupe	½ cup	7
Cherries (sour)	½ cup	9
Clementine	One	9
Cranberries	½ cup	6
Honeydew	½ cup	8
Papaya	½ cup	7
Peach	One (medium sized)	9
Pineapple	½ cup	10
Plum	One (medium sized)	8
Raspberries	½ cup	8
Strawberries	½ cup	7
Watermelon	½ cup	6

Tips and Tricks

There are plenty of other reasons besides lack of willpower that could be behind your nighttime carb cravings. Understanding why you might be reaching for the bad stuff could ease those urges, so ask yourself the following questions:

Am I starving? Some people tend to binge more on carbs at night because they're starving from not eating enough calories throughout the day. Make a point of eating something every two to three hours (preferably a mix of protein and complex carbs).

Am I tired? Eating less frequently during the day can cause your blood-sugar levels to plummet lower than usual. When that happens, your body immediately craves foods it can quickly convert into energy, and it knows that simple carbs are a fast fix.

Am I bored, sad, or stressed? Even if you don't believe that you're an emotional eater, if you find yourself raiding the fridge because you have a lot on your mind or nothing to do, look for a few alternate distractions. Tweet me (@jennawolfe) and I'll talk you right out of that fridge. Trust me, I can be a fantastic distraction. Ask my elementary school teachers.

Am I thirsty? When your body is dehydrated, it sometimes has an urge for certain foods that it knows contain water and salt. Because many processed carb-rich foods can be loaded in sodium, your body may be steering you in their direction to balance things out.

Am I due? This tip is for the ladies. Check the calendar. Many women have an increase in their metabolic rate right before their period, a spike that can sometimes cause them to naturally crave more calories. Menstruating can also cause a sudden decline in blood sugar that needs to be stabilized immediately. If that's you, either avoid temptation by keeping any foods you can't resist out of the house or answer that sugar need with a small piece of fruit.

Am I about to run a marathon? Remember, the main reason your body needs carbs is to fuel your body, so why would you give it extra gas right before bedtime when your metabolism is already slowing down for the day? Sometimes, simply reminding yourself that you're about to eat something your body doesn't need at the moment can keep an urge at bay.

The "So You Know" Science

Not all carbohydrates are created equal. All carbs raise your blood sugar to some extent, but at different levels.

Refined carbs and other simple carbs (such as fruit beverages, pretzels, chips, cakes, cookies, sodas, alcohol, white rice, regular pasta, or anything made from white flour, for example) are quickly digested into simple sugars and absorbed into your bloodstream. That surge causes your blood-sugar levels to rise, which forces your body to release a substantial amount of insulin (a hormone that can decrease how much fat your body burns and increase how much fat it stores).

On the other hand, high-quality complex carbohydrates (such as most vegetables, legumes, oatmeal, nuts and seeds, whole-grain products, and brown or wild rice) take longer to digest, are richer in fiber, and help slow the absorption of sugar into your bloodstream between meals. The end result: Your body gets a steadier stream of energy from the carbs you eat, but there's less insulin released, so you store less fat—and burn more of what's hanging on you.

Today show Tested

This Change was the hardest for Jeff Rossen to adopt. That's because the hour of 6:00 p.m. was his favorite hour of the day, mainly because of a little meal called dinner. How do I know this? Before we started, I asked him to write down his weaknesses in life. He wrote down two things: sharks and carbs—and not necessarily in that order.

A typical meal: bread, pasta, more bread, wine, another piece of bread, rice from sushi, a third piece of bread—and also a fourth piece of bread. Getting him to cut back on the carbs at night wasn't an option. Like me, he needed an all-or-nothing approach. I wasn't about to cut carbs out of his diet completely, so I had him stop at 6:00 p.m.

Did I hear about it in a text message every single night for two straight weeks? Yup—I had to increase my data plan. But then, one day, he got through dinner without wanting the bread. And the next night, it became even easier. Then a few nights later, he texted me to ask if he could stop eating carbs at 5:00 p.m. as an added challenge. With a proud tear in my eye (don't worry—it was allergies), I knew he finally got it.

This one Change saved him between 500 and 600 calories every single day. And although it was difficult for him in the beginning, the guy who literally slept with a loaf of bread under his pillow every night (not really, but only because that would make a lot of crumbs) doesn't even think about carbs anymore.

#5

Pick Two Exercises and Do Them 50 Times Throughout the Day

SIMPLY PUT...Choose any two exercises in this chapter and do 50 reps of each. It doesn't matter how long it takes you to do them, or how many you do in a row. Just do two different exercises, 50 times each, by the end of the day.

An actual conversation with my mom

MOM: Hey, Gigi!

ME: Hi, Mom. What's going on?

MOM: How can I make my tush tighter?

ME: I can put together a whole lower body workout for you.

MOM: Nah...I don't have time for that.

ME: Are you sitting down?

MOM: Umm...yes.

ME: Then stand up. Now sit back down very quietly and slowly. Now stand back up. Now sit back down. Do that fifty times while you're on the phone with me and squeeze your tush each time you stand up.

(*Less than a minute of awkward silence later…*)
MOM: OK. I did it.
ME: Mazel tov! You just found time for a workout.
MOM: (*A brief pause*) When??

No matter what you may have heard or overheard from whatever spandex-clad aerobics instructor, strength training is the key to weight loss. Let me say that again so you understand how important it is: STRENGTH TRAINING IS THE KEY TO WEIGHT LOSS. I would write it a third time, but I'm under a strict word count here, folks.

That's not based on what I've read or what I've heard others preach, it's based on what I've done myself. And it works. Strength training works your muscles and bones, burns calories, and helps your core, balance, coordination, and flexibility— all in one shot. So how awesome does strength training sound now??

OK, ladies, before you tell me you don't lift because you don't want to beef up, let me ask you this: Did Santa and the Tooth Fairy ever date? Clearly, if you believe the first myth, you probably believe the second (although the second one isn't nearly that popular).

Look, it's hard enough for men to "bulk up" by lifting weights, and they have twenty times more testosterone than women do. In other words, you won't beef up lifting weights, trust me. But what you will do is tone your muscles without building mass.

The Game Plan: Before you try some of the workout-based Changes in this book, I need your entire body prepped and ready for what's in store later. The eight multimuscle movements you're about to learn in this chapter will do just that.

Why these eight exercises? Even though there are countless moves I could have you do to get your body primed for what's ahead, these are my go-to moves. All eight of these can be done anywhere—indoors or out—and no space or equipment is needed beyond a sturdy wall (and a mat if lying down bothers your back).

For this Change, there are no tips, there are no tricks—only a few simple rules I need you to follow:

- Learn the lingo. A *repetition* or *rep* means performing an exercise one time. A *set* is a group of repetitions. For example, doing one set of 20 repetitions means you'll need to perform the exercise 20 times.

- Each day, you'll choose any two of the eight exercises in this chapter and perform them for a total of 50 reps each.
- You can do them anyway you want, so long as you complete 50 reps of each exercise before you go to bed. Want to do 1 rep every ten minutes? Fine. Feel like finishing them all off in one shot so you're done with them in a few minutes? Fantastic. I don't care how long it takes—I just want to get your body used to feeling a little burn.
- Ideally, mix and match the moves so you're not doing the same two every day. You'll target more muscles and your body will be even more prepared later on.
- Finally, continue doing two exercises each day until you reach Change #10. (That's when your first full-body workout will begin.)

THE EXERCISES

Apple Pickers

SETUP: Stand straight with your feet shoulder-width apart and your arms extended up over your head.

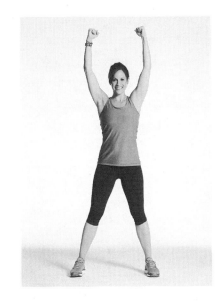

THE MOTION: Pull your elbows down as you bring your right knee up toward your chest as high as you can. Bring yourself back to the setup position (arms above you with both feet on the floor) and repeat, this time by raising your left knee up as you pull your elbows down. Lifting your right knee, then your left, counts as 1 rep.

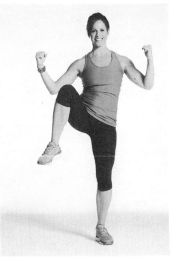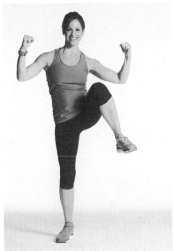

Too challenging? Raise each knee up only to about your waist.

Too easy? Hold a light dumbbell in each hand to add some extra resistance.

Crab Kicks

SETUP: Get into a tabletop position by sitting down and placing both your hands and feet on the floor. Your heels should be beneath your knees, palms underneath your shoulders, with your butt raised off the floor.

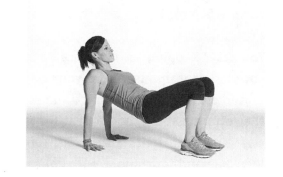

THE MOTION: Keeping your balance, quickly extend your left leg straight out in front of you. Your left foot should end up about the same level as your head or slightly higher, depending on your flexibility and coordination. Quickly bring your left leg back down to the setup position as you simultaneously extend your right leg straight out in front of you. (That's 1 rep.) Continue alternating from left to right for the entire exercise.

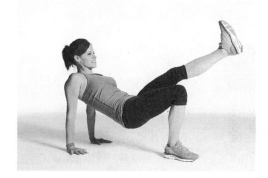

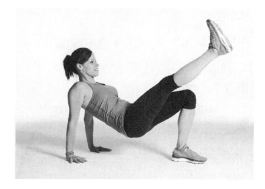

Too challenging? Keeping your hands and feet on the floor, just sit and pulse your butt up and down (without letting it touch the floor) for twenty-five reps. Rest for five seconds, then pulse again for another twenty-five reps.

Too easy? Keeping your balance, quickly swing your left foot up just above your right knee and touch it with your right hand. Return to the setup position, then repeat the move by swinging your right foot up just above your left knee and touching it with your left hand. (That's 1 rep.)

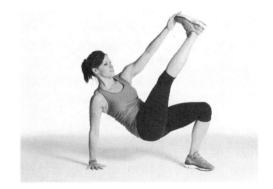

Hip Raises

SETUP: Lie flat on your back on a mat (or carpeted floor) with your knees bent. Your feet should be flat on the floor and spaced shoulder-width apart. Extend your arms out along your sides.

THE MOTION: Squeeze your glutes as you press down through your heels and slowly lift your hips toward the ceiling. Stop once your body forms a straight line from your knees down to your shoulders, then slowly lower yourself back down to the floor. (That's 1 rep.)

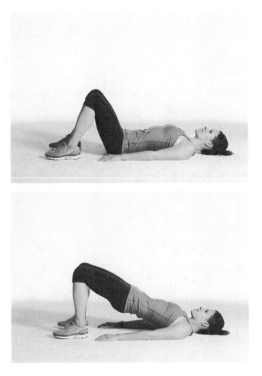

Too challenging? Raise your hips only as high as you comfortably can, even if it's only a few inches.

Too easy? Cross your arms over your chest, extend your right leg up toward the ceiling, then hold it there as you perform the exercise using your left leg only. After performing the required number of reps, switch positions— left leg up, right foot on the floor—and repeat for the required number of reps.

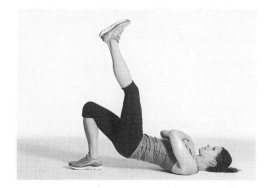

Pikes

SETUP: Get in a push-up position—legs extended behind you, feet together, with your weight on your toes.

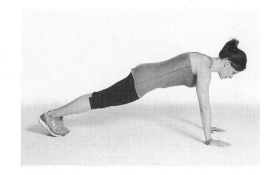

THE MOTION: Keeping your hands on the floor, quickly spring off your toes and hop forward to bring your feet closer to your hands. (Your body will look like an upside-down V from the side.) Quickly hop back to the setup position. (That's 1 rep.)

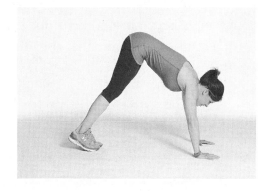

Too challenging? Just hop your feet a few inches toward your hands.

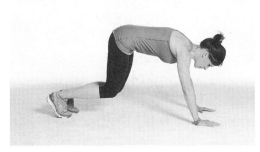

Too easy? In between pikes, do a push-up.

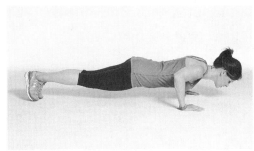

Mountain Climbers (Slow and Fast)

SETUP: Get in a push-up position by placing your hands on the floor shoulder-width apart and extending your legs behind you with your weight on your toes. Your body should form a straight line from your head to your heels.

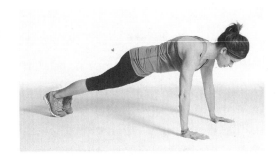

THE MOTION:

For Slow Mountain Climbers: Once you're balanced, lift your right foot off the floor and slowly bring your right knee toward your chest without your foot touching the floor. Reverse the move so that your right foot is back on the floor and repeat, this time by slowly bringing your left knee toward your chest. (That's 1 rep.)

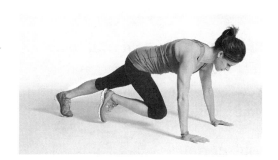

For Fast Mountain Climbers: Follow the same instructions as above, but perform the exercise as quickly as possible *without* sacrificing your form.

Too challenging? Do a plank knee touch. Instead of lifting each foot and bringing your knees forward, keep your feet on the floor and alternate touching each knee to the floor.

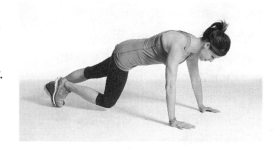

Too easy? Instead of keeping your hands shoulder-width apart, bring your hands together so that your pointer fingers and thumbs touch each other.

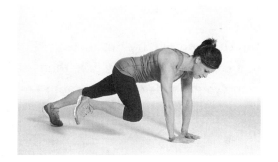

Squats

SETUP: Stand straight with your feet shoulder-width apart and your arms hanging down by your sides.

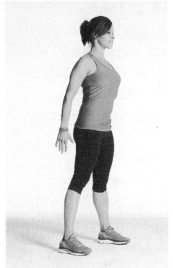 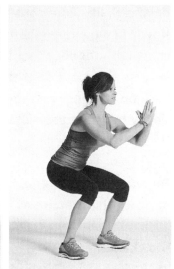

THE MOTION: Keeping your head and back straight, slowly squat down until your thighs are parallel to the floor, bringing your arms in front of your body, palms together. Don't move your feet, so you really engage your legs, glutes, and core. Push yourself back up into the setup position. (That's 1 rep.) Try to take two seconds to lower yourself down and two seconds to push back up.

Too challenging? Try this instead: Sit down in a chair or on a sturdy box, then—without using your hands or moving your feet—stand. Next, sit down slowly so that you don't make a sound, and repeat.

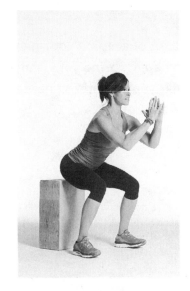

Too easy? Repeat the exercise as described, only each time you squat down, pause for three seconds in the down position before slowly standing back up.

Toy Soldiers

SETUP: Stand straight with your feet hip-width apart and your arms extended straight in front of you, palms facing down.

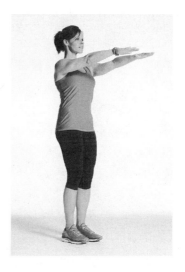

THE MOTION: Keeping your arms parallel to the floor and legs as straight as possible, bring your right leg up in front of you—the goal is to try to touch your toes to the middle of your right palm. Bring your right leg back down and repeat, this time by bringing your left leg up and trying to touch your toes to your left palm. (That's 1 rep.)

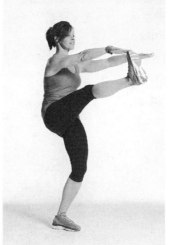
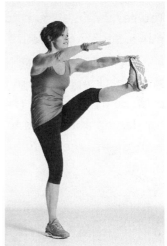

Too challenging? Instead of raising each leg to touch your toes to your palms, bend and lift each knee up toward your arms.

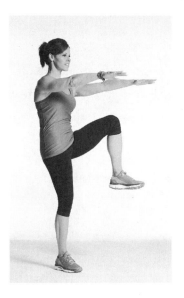

Too easy? Add a squat to the move. Squat until your thighs are parallel to the floor. As you stand back up, perform the exercise as described (swinging one leg up and trying to touch your toes to the middle of your palm).

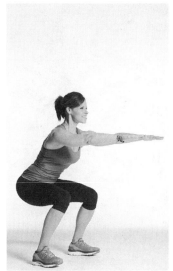
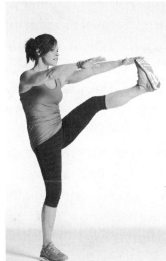

Wall Push-Offs

SETUP: Stand about three to four feet in front of a sturdy wall and extend your arms in front of you at shoulder level. Lean forward and place your palms flat on the wall, hands shoulder-width apart. (Your body should now be at a slight angle with your arms straight.) Keeping your back flat (don't arch forward), bend your elbows and slowly bring your chest as close to the wall as possible. Don't worry if your heels lift off the floor so you're resting on the balls of your feet—that's normal.

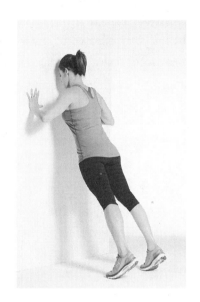

THE MOTION: Push yourself away from the wall until your arms are extended, hands lifted just off the wall. (That's 1 rep.) Place your hands back on the wall and repeat.

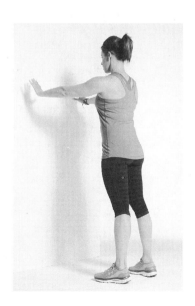

Too challenging? Move your feet a few inches closer to the wall to make the angle of the move easier.

Too easy? Try a kneeling push-up position instead. Place your hands on the floor about shoulder-width apart, bend your elbows to lower yourself to the floor, then press yourself back up.

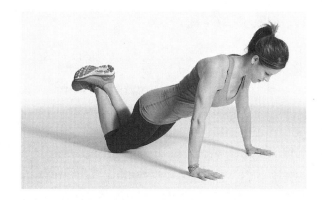

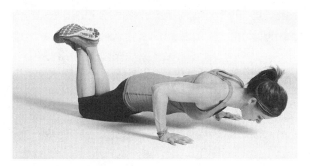

Still too easy?
If that's still a breeze, you're ready for a regular push-up. (Get off your knees so you're up on your toes and follow the same up-down directions.)

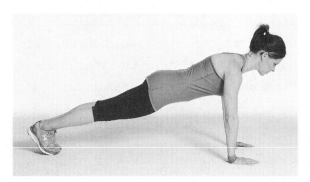

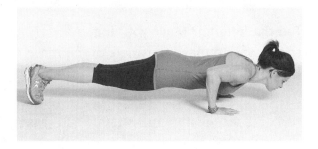

The "So You Know" Science

I hate to break it to you, but once you hit thirty, your body starts to lose muscle at a rate of 3 to 5 percent every decade. Maybe you think you wouldn't miss that amount of muscle, but it's a deficit that causes your metabolism to slow down, burn fewer calories, and store more of whatever calories you're eating as unwanted fat. Doing some form of regular resistance training can prevent that from happening and, according to the CDC,[1] raise your metabolism by as much as 15 percent.

Beyond keeping your metabolism revved and your muscles right where you like them, resistance training also plays a key role in preventing calcium loss, strengthening your bones, and improving your overall balance. More importantly, it can even make you less likely to have to deal with metabolic syndrome, a cluster of five factors—ranging from having a large waist to high blood pressure—that have been shown to increase your risk of developing heart disease and diabetes.

#6
Redo How You Chew

SIMPLY PUT . . . Do these three things every time you eat a meal:

1. When you take a bite of food, chew a minimum of twenty times before swallowing.
2. Take a sip of water after every bite.
3. Once your plate is empty, wait twenty minutes before going back for seconds.

Why It Works: Chewing twenty times before swallowing may be difficult if you've chosen to eat apple sauce for lunch or yogurt or pudding (but please . . . don't eat pudding for lunch), but it'll definitely keep you from overeating.

Keep in mind it takes about twenty minutes for your stomach to tell your brain it's full so it can flip off your hunger switch. And in those twenty minutes, you could do so much damage throwing back excess calories.

So how do you slow it down? It's time to really think about chewing your food. A lot of people mindlessly take a bite and swallow it in three chews—and I'm probably being generous with that number! But when you take the time to chew your food at least twenty times before you swallow, you'll give your brain the time it needs to catch up. Sure, it might take you three hours to finish lunch, but consider it "me" time...Or forget about me, consider it "you" time.

Slowing down your eating pace with all those extra chews will also make you more aware of what you're eating. Bad processed foods earn their reputation as junk (is that a technical term?) because there's usually nothing of value in them. No fiber, no nutrients—nothing but surplus calories and shame. (They won't list *shame* in the ingredients, but it's there. Trust me.)

When you chew junk food for a longer period of time, that point really hits home. Good luck getting to twenty, because without anything of substance inside them, the bad stuff typically disintegrates in your mouth, which is usually why we go back for more. But nutrient-dense, high-fiber foods that have more to offer take time to gnash. Before you know it, you'll be gaining a deeper understanding of the foods you're eating—and may find yourself making smarter choices—simply by taking the time to get to know them better.

DON'T STOP THERE...

I'm sure you've heard the advice, *never finish all the food on your plate*. Well, that may work for you, but it's never worked for me. I love food. I look forward to eating food. I love the satisfying feeling of finishing every ounce of food on my plate (OK, you get the idea). But since this is great advice, I had to adjust.

When I got pregnant with my first daughter, Harper, my only true craving was cold cereal. Not pizza or ice cream or Hot Pockets, but cold cereal. I couldn't be left alone in the cereal aisle at the supermarket for fear I'd never get home. Narrowing down my choices to three or four boxes was like being asked to choose which child I loved most. I literally wanted everything off every shelf. From Cheerios to Fruity Pebbles to Bran Flakes, Cookie Crisp, Apple Jacks, Total, Honeycomb, even Grape-Nuts. And don't get me started on Cinnamon Toast Crunch.

There was something about the sound of the flakes hitting the bowl, the swish of the cold milk joining in, and the throwback to my youth as I sat with my pregnant belly and devoured my morning (and midmorning and afternoon and midafternoon and oftentimes early evening) crunch.

Do you know what the *Today* show gave me as a going-away present when I went on maternity leave? Not flowers or candy or bibs. They gave me cereal. Remember those adorable little travel packs they'd sell bunched together and wrapped in cellophane? The ones that were sold as one serving per box but everyone could eat all eight boxes at once? Yeah, well, the *Today* show wrapped up about sixty of them for me. Excessive? Hardly. I could have eaten sixty-one.

So the way I saw it, I had two choices: Put on an extra twenty pounds or adjust my craving. I had to choose option B. Here's what I did: Instead of the big bowl I wanted every morning, I compromised and ate my guilty pleasure only out of a small coffee mug, reducing the amount I was eating per serving by almost half.

Using smaller plates and bowls (and thinner, taller glasses) makes it feel like you've eaten and drunk more than you really have. What that really does is force you to serve up smaller portions. In fact, a few scientists with time on their hands already figured out that swapping larger plates for a medium-sized dish (about eight or nine inches in diameter) causes most people to consume roughly 20 percent less food.

Once your plate, bowl, coffee mug, kiddie cup (whatever you choose to downsize to) is empty, then wait a few minutes. If you're still hungry after twenty minutes, then I won't stop you from going back for seconds.

Twenty minutes may seem like an eternity for you—especially after you've already managed to eat more slowly by chewing more—and I get that. But just try it for three days and trust in the system. You'll be so surprised, because you won't be going back for seconds as often as you think. Your body will begin to adjust itself automatically, and within a few days you'll begin to realize that you're never as hungry as you think you are.

Tips and Tricks

Chewing longer and choosing smaller-sized plates aren't the only ways you can give your brain enough time to register how full you really are. Here are some other handy tips:

Put your fork or spoon down between bites. Holding that utensil in your hand only makes it easier to unconsciously stab or scoop up another taste, even if you may not really be ready for another bite.

Slice and dice your food as small as possible. Not only does cutting up your food into tinier portions give your stomach more time to talk to your brain, research has shown it may actually trick your brain into believing you're eating more by giving what's on your plate more volume.

Go bold. When the color of your food matches your dinnerware, you tend to pack on more of it. Instead, pick plates and bowls that are a contrast to whatever it is you're eating, so your meal never blends into the background.

Pick up two sticks instead. Using a pair of chopsticks may be challenging, but that's the idea. Not only do they force you to eat smaller portions, but all that precision makes it even harder to eat faster than you should.

Lend a hand when it's time for dinner. Whenever you're dining with others, offer to set the table. That will give you more control over dropping a plate, bowl, or glass where you're seated that's slightly smaller than everyone else's at the table.

Eat everything in reverse. Instead of just digging into your main course, change the order of how you nibble. Start with the healthiest food on your plate, then work your way around your plate from most healthy to least healthy. That way, if you get full before clearing your plate, anything left on it will most likely be something you shouldn't be eating too much of in the first place.

Make your dentist proud. Who *really* brushes after every meal? Well, now you do! Having fresh minty breath makes it a little easier to resist snacking so soon between meals, and peppermint is also a natural appetite suppressant. I didn't believe this worked until I tried it for a week. As soon as I ate my last bite of dinner, I brushed my teeth. It immediately curbed my appetite for dessert and for a late snack. Call me lazy, but the thought of having to brush my teeth again (along with the fresh minty taste in my mouth) kept me in check.

Try to munch only when you're mellow. If you're racing to eat because you have no time, your body's already under stress—not a good place to be in, because stress shuts down digestion. Instead, try to schedule more time for your meals and snacks so that everything you eat gets broken down more efficiently.

Use a dish—not your digits. Sneaking a handful of food from the fridge or a box or bag in your pantry adds up if you never keep track. But it's much harder to eat mindlessly if you always use a plate or bowl.

Grab a seat whenever you eat. Walking while you eat makes you less conscious of what you're eating, so plant it. Just avoid sitting and eating in front of anything that may steal your attention away (the TV, your computer or tablet, a movie screen, etc.).

Never dine where it's dim or dark. The lower the lighting, the easier it is to ignore what you're putting into your mouth. It may also leave you feeling more relaxed, which can lower your inhibitions and leave you more likely to snack away.

Turn your back to your food. Try not to sit facing either the kitchen or serving area if you can help it. Research has shown that those more in control of their weight tend to sit with their backs to their food. That goes for putting serving plates or bowls on the table too. The more food that's placed in front of you, the more likely you'll be to reach for another helping, so keep any extra food on the stove or kitchen counter.

Surround yourself with appetite-curbing colors. Seeing green, orange, red, and yellow objects seems to stimulate appetite more than being around blue, black, and brown objects, which tend to be more appetite-suppressing colors. That doesn't mean you have to repaint! Just rethinking the color of your tableware—including your plates, napkins, glassware, placemats, and table runner—can subdue your eating habits.

CHANGE

#7
Adjust Your Expectations

SIMPLY PUT . . . From today on, I want you to say the following three things each morning. Say them as a promise, as a reminder, as motivation. Say them out loud:

1. "Life begins at the end of your comfort zone."
2. "If it doesn't challenge you, it won't change you."
3. "We can't become what we want to be by remaining who we are."

Welcome to quitting time.

This is when the weak stop and the strong persevere. It's also why many of the people around you (and for that matter, two-thirds of US adults over age twenty) are still overweight, no matter how badly they want to do something about it.

If you've been using this book as a thirty-day program, then you're already one week into the plan. And if it's taken you a little longer to get here because you've allowed each Change to really sink in and become part of you, then listen up.

As the health/fitness correspondent for the *Today* show, I was assigned a month-long series to convert one of my colleagues, Jeff Rossen, from fair to fit.

I was to put him on a plan, get him to the gym, videotape his (almost) every move, and then sit back and watch the pounds roll off. It was going to make for sensational TV. There was just one problem—his body wasn't quite on the same time frame that we were.

A little background first: Rossen had never been to the gym—ever. He never played sports, although he did touch a signed NBA basketball one time at an auction (but it was still in the glass case). He never met a carbohydrate he didn't like. (Nice to meet you, loaf of bread. Is that your cousin, second loaf?) And he never ever thought he'd be able to stick to an eating and exercise plan.

Good luck to me, right?

But give the guy credit because he was committed to it. So he signed up, agreed to follow every last direction and guideline of mine, and was ready to work. I didn't throw him in the deep end, much in the same way I didn't start this book with a killer workout. We made some early, manageable changes, such as reducing his afternoon and nighttime intake of carbs, implementing a 10k-step-a-day program, and increasing his water intake—all of the things you're now doing through this book.

Rossen wanted to lose about fifteen pounds in one month. He thought he'd lose at least fourteen by Day Two. I tried to temper his expectations, but he was sure that if he did everything I instructed him to do, he'd shed weight immediately. Unfortunately, weight loss doesn't work that way. Everyone's body is built differently and runs differently. What might take a week for one person to start dropping weight may take three or four weeks for someone else.

That being said, after three weeks he had lost only four pounds and was tempted to quit. Why put himself through all this for such measly results, he wondered. I received text after text questioning the plan, his body, the whole program—and each was met with the same answers: "Be patient." "You didn't gain this weight in a week, and you won't lose it in a week." "You're doing all the right things." "Give your body a chance to figure out what you're asking it to do."

"Trust me."

By the fourth week, the weight starting falling off, and by the end of our month-long series, he had lost close to thirteen pounds and dropped two belt notches. He was thrilled. I was thrilled. His belt was thrilled.

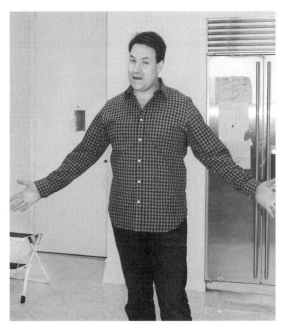

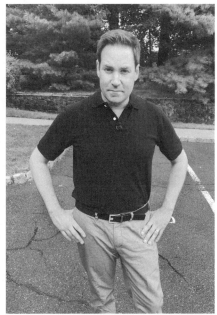

Jeff, then   Jeff, today

Losing weight slowly is a good thing. And right now, I want you to forget what you think you know about weight loss, getting in shape, and improving your overall health.

The fact is, when you take weight off too quickly (which many fad diets try to do by cutting out entire food groups or restricting calories below healthy standards), your body's homeostatic mechanisms go into defense mode. In a nutshell, your body thinks that it's starving, so it tries to protect you by lowering your metabolism to a slow crawl to conserve calories. It's a sweet gesture (and a natural survival strategy), but it brings any effort you make moving forward to lose weight through exercise and being smart about your diet to a grinding halt.

You need to have patience. That was the agreement we made before all of this started, remember? This is a system. This is a process. And most important, this is the way it works—the way it has always worked—and we are doing this slowly because you want to do it correctly. And you need to trust me when I say that there's a switch in you that's about to be flipped.

If you're extremely lucky, it's already happened for you. But for most people, it takes a bit longer before that switch gets flipped. It never happens at the exact same moment for everyone, even if you and a friend have started this journey with me together. It doesn't happen at the exact same time for my clients either. But somewhere along the thirty Changes, it's going to happen to you, and when it does, once that switch is flipped, you'll arrive at a whole new mindset.

Every Change you've embraced prior, and every new Change you're about to make moving forward, will suddenly become easier and require less effort. I can't promise you that you won't flip that switch until after all thirty Changes become a part of your life, but when it clicks, it clicks. And all this work you've been doing that once felt like labor will soon feel like a lifestyle.

DON'T STOP THERE...

There are three factors that help us make a change in our lives: muscle, mind, and heart.

We always start with our muscles. They're big and strong and require less thinking and more doing. So we muscle our way through a workout or an all-nighter study session or a work deadline. But eventually our bodies—specifically our muscles—begin to tire out, and that's when I want you to use your mind. Your mind will carry you over matter. Your mind will take you past the discomfort of the workouts, past the annoyances of eating clean, and past the desire to quit.

But when your mind goes soft, when you know each Change is important but you still find yourself wanting to quit, that's when I want your heart to take over and push you through. It's time to look in the mirror and say, "I may not see results yet, but I know in my heart that I'm doing the right thing and that eventually this will all lead to something great."

Muscle, mind, and heart.

And you have to keep telling yourself that. That's why, every morning, I want you to put down that glass of water after you've taken your twenty sips from it and say these three things to yourself:

1. "Life begins at the end of your comfort zone."
2. "If it doesn't challenge you, it won't change you."
3. "We can't become what we want to be by remaining who we are."

Saying those words aloud is you telling yourself that every single choice you make moving forward may be a conscious and difficult choice—and it may be work—but it's worth it. It reminds you that you don't want to go back to the way it was or the person you used to hate seeing in the mirror.

Tips and Tricks

If this journey was an easy one, everyone would be doing it. You may not be everyone, but you *are* the one who will look, feel, sleep, move, eat, act, and *be* better a month from now. Using a few of these recommendations could make that journey a little more effortless.

Play back your past failures. The next time you find yourself making an excuse not to stick with any Change you've learned (and will learn) from this book, replay those moments in the past when you skipped a workout, overate, or quit a diet. Remind yourself how giving in led you here, then use that feeling to prevent yourself from repeating a failure in the future.

This lifestyle isn't just for the workweek. That means that weekends count. Being good with your Changes all week long may make you feel you can be more lax on the weekends. But start slacking off from Friday night through Sunday night and you've just wasted a third of your week being bad. Instead, anticipate that the weekends will be way more tempting for you and try to plan accordingly.

Make a "worth the time" list. You already know which achievements were worth every ounce of your effort, from getting your master's degree or having your first child to growing out your bangs and suffering through a fourteen-hour flight for a fantastic vacation. So write down a list of things that took time but were worth it in the end—and realize that soon, adopting these thirty Changes will make that list.

Never lose sleep over a setback. Will you forget to send your food diary one night or wake up without having your twenty sips the next morning? Maybe, but when it happens, don't beat yourself up. Most people react to slipping by throwing in the towel or telling themselves they'll try again tomorrow or next week. Instead, move on as soon as you mess up.

Ask yourself, "Is this really that difficult?" You could be exaggerating how hard a Change is, just to justify not doing it as often. To keep yourself from blowing things out of proportion, measure how inconvenient a Change might be against other struggles you've overcome that were much harder.

Remember the time that you've lost. If losing weight at a healthy pace of about one pound each week seems slow, count up how many weeks you've been at your current weight. Each one of those weeks represents a week you could have been one pound less than the week before.

Imagine your future you. At the end of the day, take five minutes to close your eyes and picture how you'll look and feel when your goals are met. Think of the things you'll be able to do more easily, or maybe even for the first time. You need to visualize who you will eventually become at the end of this journey and remind yourself that every ounce of hard work you put in that day will soon be worth it.

Eat Your Fast Food (no, obviously not that fast food!)

SIMPLY PUT . . . Do this every three days:

1. Find the best fresh fruits and vegetables you can.
2. Cut them up into easy-to-grab pieces.
3. Place all the pieces in two huge bowls (fruit in one bowl and veggies in the other) and pop them in the fridge.

I know what you're thinking . . .

"Really? Eating my fruits and veggies is worthy of its own chapter? What's next, no cotton candy for breakfast??"

Yes, fruits and veggies are worthy of a chapter and here's why. It's not about what you eat—it's about what you don't eat. When I'm hungry, I need to eat immediately. If I want a snack, I want that snack yesterday. So I'll open my fridge and grab the first thing that I find. What ends up inhaled has little to do with taste or nutrition. Instead, it's all about access.

So put the best food you can find right in front of your face and I guarantee you'll eat it.

I'm willing to bet you're just like me, especially at the end of the day when you're tired, you're trying to pull together dinner, and the willpower you had in the morning has crashed to an all-time low. Hit the fridge in that state when hunger strikes, and odds are you'll eat the first thing you see. One night, I literally ate three forkfuls of sauerkraut because it was there…At least, I *think* that was sauerkraut. I really hope it was sauerkraut.

We're like children that way. All we want is whatever's easy and accessible. And let's face it: If we were any better than that, there would be no such thing as fast food. There wouldn't be an entire billion-dollar industry dedicated to letting us pull up, pay up, and pig out. So why not plan for that eating onslaught by always having something healthy that's just as easy and accessible?

So buy three days' worth of fruit and veggies (after that, they get lazy and start going bad), slice and dice them into bite-size pieces, throw it all into two bowls, and you're done. All that food is bright, it's colorful, and it's now the closest thing to your hands the next time you find yourself speed-dating your icebox for a snack. I also keep some low-fat cheese, hummus, and a jar of almond butter in the fridge all the time to help turn my quick little snack into something more filling, nutritious, and tasty.

DON'T STOP THERE…

There are "A" fruits, there are "B" fruits, and then there are "C" fruits, so let's go all the way. No offense, honeydew and cantaloupe, but everyone knows you're always the last two left in any hospital or airplane fruit salad. Instead, treat yourself to the "A" fruits because that's what you deserve—the good stuff like blueberries, strawberries, pomegranate seeds, pineapple chunks, and watermelon—then throw in some mint leaves and make it inviting. Instead of just turning that big bowl of fruit into something handy, shape it into something you would see at a party and can't wait to attack.

The same rules apply to your veggies. I'm not against celery and cucumbers, because they're seriously low in calories and packed with water and a little fiber that can help you feel fuller. But in the nutrient department, they rank right up there with iceberg lettuce in their nutritional near-worthlessness.

A-Lister Eats to Include

Apples, strawberries, mangoes, rich red grapes, peaches, and watermelon are all fine choices, but they aren't the only ones with something to bring to the table.

Bananas: Not only are they a great source of fiber, they're also teeming with potassium, a nutrient that helps prevent muscle cramps, stimulates the formation of red blood cells, and aids in regulating blood pressure.

Blackberries: Just a cup contains close to eight grams of fiber (almost 30 percent of the amount people should be eating each day but never bother to). The phytonutrients and antioxidants in blackberries (particularly one known as anthocyanin) may also help slow down the decline in brain function and reverse memory loss associated with aging.[1]

Blueberries: Loaded with more vitamins, minerals, and fiber per ounce than practically any other piece of fruit out there, blueberries also contain anthocyanin.

Broccoli: The green giant known for lowering the risk of heart disease is loaded with iron, calcium, fiber, beta-carotene, and a phytochemical called sulforaphane, a potent compound that helps fight cancer and osteoarthritis. [2,3]

Carrots: Not only is the root veggie a good source of fiber and potassium, carrots are bursting with beta-carotene, an antioxidant that may help prevent arthritis, promote eye health, and improve your skin.[4]

Cauliflower: Among its many benefits, this cruciferous veggie ranks second (only broccoli beats it) in having the highest saturation of glucosinolates, which help your body detoxify and could aid in cancer prevention.[5]

Cherries: Packed with vitamin C and fiber, they also contain anthocyanin, an antioxidant associated with reducing inflammation.[6]

Cherry tomatoes: High in vitamin B6 and folate, they also contain lycopene, a powerful antioxidant linked with lowering your risk of stroke[7] and eliminating dangerous free radicals that can damage your DNA.[8]

Citrus fruits: From blood oranges and grapefruit to kumquats and tangerines, all are good sources of fiber, vitamin C, and flavonoids that can protect you against heart-related diseases.[9]

Cranberries: If you have a taste for eating them fresh, this antioxidant-rich fruit has been shown to increase your HDL (the "good" cholesterol).[10] And they're antibacterial, which is why they're so effective in treating and preventing urinary tract infections.[11]

Kiwifruit: Fibrous and fortified with vitamin C (250 percent of the RDA for the nutrient is in one cup alone), the fuzzy fruit is also a significant source of potassium and vitamin E.

Papayas: Beyond the assortment of vitamins it offers (A, C, and E, to name a few), the tropical fruit also contains zeaxanthin, an antioxidant that filters harmful blue light rays and may ward off damage from macular degeneration.[12]

Pears: With its skin intact, this fruit contains a full five grams of soluble fiber in just one medium-sized pear, which can significantly help reduce blood cholesterol levels and prevent heart disease.[13,14]

Pineapples: The tropical fruit isn't just sweet tasting, it's got vitamin C and manganese, which may reduce PMS symptoms.[15]

Pomegranates: All the effort of opening one is worth it. Beyond being abundant in vitamin C, it's full of antioxidants, including tannins, which may protect your heart.[16]

Plums and apricots: Brimming with vitamins A and C, both have a decent amount of anthocyanin and potassium.

Raspberries: Just like blackberries, raspberries offer plenty of fiber and antioxidants, including ellagic acid, which seems to have some anti-cancer properties.[17]

Red bell peppers: Despite the orange's reputation for being the vitamin C king, this veggie has about three times the amount. Plus, they contain ample amounts of vitamins A and E, which can promote joint, skin, and eye health.[18]

Sugar snap peas: Within all that crunchiness hides a decent amount of folate (for your heart), vitamins B6 and K (for your bones), and even a little iron to help prevent anemia and fatigue.

Zucchini: Low in calories (a medium-sized one is only about 30-plus calories) and filled with water, zucchini will surprise your body with both lutein and zeaxanthin,[19] two phytonutrients that promote healthy eyesight.[20]

Tips and Tricks

It really doesn't get any simpler than asking you to cut up two bowls of fruits and vegetables, does it? Still, there are a handful of things you can try to make this Change either easier or more effective.

Go for the brightest in the bunch. The richer and brighter a vegetable is (whether it's bright green, orange, red, or yellow), the more nutritionally dense it's likely to be. So when you shop, don't just grab whatever's fresh, but step back from the display to see which pieces really catch your eye. You'll get more nutritional bang for the same buck.

Get someone else to slice it. You'll blow a few bucks on bad foods, so splurge a little for prewashed, precut fruits and veggies if it saves you time and makes you more likely to make this Change.

The canned kind does not count. Canned fruits and vegetables are typically high in preservatives, particularly sugar (with fruits) and sodium (with vegetables). Although they may make things easier in a pinch, skip them for something fresh.

Switch in one new food each week. Every fruit and vegetable has its own unique mix of nutrients, and like snowflakes and Baldwin brothers, no two are exactly the same. To keep your taste buds guessing and your body exposed to a wider variety of vitamins and minerals, force yourself to try at least one new fruit or vegetable every week.

Veg out in the morning. Most people wait until lunch or dinner before eating vegetables, so look for ways to grab some of the veggies in your bowl and stick some into your morning meals.

The "So You Know" Science

Yes, fresh fruits and vegetables are a tremendous natural source of fiber, vitamins, minerals, antioxidants, and other nutrients. And could I list them all from vitamin A to zinc and fill every page of this book? I could—but would you honestly read it? Thought not.

I could tell you that according to the Centers for Disease Control and Prevention (CDC), a healthy diet rich in fruits and veggies may reduce the risk of cancer and other chronic diseases. But you're not an idiot. You know that already.

However, something you might not know is that the amount of fruits and vegetables you should eat each day depends on your age, sex, and activity level. Even though following my thirty Changes will most likely leave you hitting that mark daily without having to try or think about it, this will give you an idea of how much of each is ideal:

LADIES			
If you're...	and your activity level every day is...	you should be eating this many cups of fruit daily...	and you should be eating this many cups of vegetables daily...
25	less than 30 minutes	2	2.5
25	30 to 60 minutes	2	3
25	more than 60 minutes	2	3
35	less than 30 minutes	1.5	2.5
35	30 to 60 minutes	2	2.5
35	more than 60 minutes	2	3
45	less than 30 minutes	1.5	2.5
45	30 to 60 minutes	2	2.5
45	more than 60 minutes	2	3
55	less than 30 minutes	1.5	2
55	30 to 60 minutes	1.5	2.5
55	more than 60 minutes	2	3

... AND GENTLEMEN			
If you're...	and your activity level every day is...	you should be eating this many cups of fruit daily...	and you should be eating this many cups of veggies daily...
25	less than 30 minutes	2	3
25	30 to 60 minutes	2.5	3.5
25	more than 60 minutes	2.5	4
35	less than 30 minutes	2	3
35	30 to 60 minutes	2	3.5
35	more than 60 minutes	2.5	4
45	less than 30 minutes	2	3
45	30 to 60 minutes	2	3.5
45	more than 60 minutes	2.5	3.5
55	less than 30 minutes	2	3
55	30 to 60 minutes	2	3.5
55	more than 60 minutes	2.5	3.5

Stop, Sit, and Disengage for at Least Five Minutes a Day

SIMPLY PUT . . . At some point each day:

1. Step away from whatever it is you're doing.
2. Find a nice quiet place where no one can bother you.
3. Sit, close your eyes, and think about nothing for at least five minutes.

Five minutes.

That's it.

If you consider that you're awake on average about fifteen hours a day, that's nine hundred minutes. Surely you can find five of those to call your very own. I'll admit, it can be hard in the beginning if you're used to running around all day. The first time I tried it, I put every ounce of effort I had into finding my inner calm. When I literally couldn't sit still any longer, I called it a session and fully expected to have reached somewhere near five minutes.

It was thirty-nine seconds.

It's no secret that I speak fast and I move fast, and if I'm not careful, I react fast. But if I don't pause for five minutes and just take it all in, whether it's just to look out the window or close my eyes and let myself mindlessly drift off to somewhere else, it gets to be too much. It's because you never realize how fast you're going until you stop for a second, just like you can't comprehend how loud your life is until you take the time to quiet it down.

Five minutes—that's really all I need. It's my very own self-imposed time-out. It sort of brings it all back so I can start from scratch and begin moving again.

Even if you're not the kind of person that goes from zero to one hundred, you need to acknowledge how incredibly busy you get between your ears. You have to try to settle the soul down a little bit. It's a small break that sheds stress and gives back so much, yet surprisingly few people bother to try it.

When you let yourself stay stressed, your body takes it out on you in countless ways. Headaches, bad skin, digestion problems, and insomnia are at one end of that spectrum, while heart issues, premature aging, a lower sex drive, and chronic back pain sit on the other.

Stress also causes your adrenal glands to release cortisol, which not only raises things you don't want breaking records (like your blood pressure and blood sugar), it also makes your fat cells bigger and even causes your body to store more body fat.

The 10,000 steps you're already putting in each day, plus the strength training you started with Change #5, will go a long way toward reducing stress. But just stepping back and out for five minutes—especially during those moments when your brain and body need it most—will be your greatest ally when it comes to eliminating stress on the spot.

My Five-Minute Formula

Disengaging for five minutes doesn't mean turning on the TV, sitting down to go through your e-mails, or checking your Facebook, Instagram, and Twitter accounts.

Disengaging is disengaging.

It's all about doing absolutely nothing but quieting your mind, relaxing your muscles, and just sitting in a state of nothingness for five whole minutes. It's time spent being alone with yourself and, to be honest, it's probably the only time aside from being asleep that you ever get to do that over the entire course of the day.

But for something so seemingly effortless and quick, stopping and doing *absolutely nothing* can be extremely difficult for most people. Here are the basics to help pull it off:

1. Plop down somewhere quiet, preferably a place where nothing else is going on. No one should be able to talk to you, and nothing should be around that could stimulate you. That means no computer or tablet, no TV, no music in the background, no phone that may vibrate, not a single person that could bother you—nothing!

2. Set a timer for six minutes. Why six? Because I want you to disengage for a full five minutes and I don't want you to waste any of that valuable time getting yourself into the zone you need to be in. Also, if you're like me, the first few times you do this, you'll spend that whole last minute looking at the timer to see if you set it right, because it'll seem way longer than five minutes. Yes, I realize that defeats the entire purpose. Just know that eventually this Change caught on with me and I now do this every single day.

3. Sit comfortably with your hands on your lap (or whatever feels natural to you), close your eyes, and just let your body relax. Imagine melting into your chair like a candle.

4. Concentrate on breathing in through your nose and out through your mouth as slowly and evenly as possible. Be aware of your breathing, making each breath not too deep and not too shallow, but don't count how many seconds it takes you to fill your lungs and release—that's work!

5. Clear your mind of everything and don't worry if you're doing it right. The more you practice, the more relaxed you'll be the next time.

DON'T STOP THERE...

Feel like going beyond five minutes, or putting your life on pause more often than just once a day? If you have the time, do it.

The same goes for allowing yourself a nap when you need one and getting an extra hour of sleep each night. Between two little kids and a crazy job, I'm definitely guilty of not getting enough sleep, so I'm the last person to tell you to sleep more. That's why I didn't make it one of my thirty Changes. If it's something I can't manage every day myself, I'd be a hypocrite to make you do it.

But here's the deal: When I can sneak in an afternoon nap, I do. A quick nap not only helps remove stress, but it can help reduce fatigue and improve your alertness and memory.

A lack of sleep can affect a running list of functions in your body. Need a list? Here's a short one: Being sleep-deprived impairs your memory and logical reasoning, increases your risk of developing a chronic health condition, slows down your metabolism, and boosts the stress hormone cortisol, so you burn fewer calories and store many more.

So how much sleep is enough? Although researchers haven't pinpointed the exact amount, if you're between the ages of twenty-six and sixty-four, it's recommended that you snooze from seven to nine hours a day—give or take. So give it a try—seriously, don't let me stop you.

Tips and Tricks

Whether you're looking to tune out for five minutes, take a nap for twenty, or tweak your typical eight-hour nocturnal stretch, these cues can help you make the most out of every second you snooze.

Take your pulse to tune out. Looking for another way to lose yourself beyond your breathing? Try placing your hands on your lap and lightly press your fingers on your wrist so you can feel your pulse. Don't count beats—just let yourself be aware of your heartbeat as you relax.

Travel somewhere nice in your mind. Keeping your eyes closed, use your imagination and try to create the most relaxing place possible. As you do, don't just see it but try to imagine how the environment feels, sounds, and smells, whether it's a crisp breeze coming down off the mountaintop or the salty air wafting from the surf.

Stare at the center. Even with your eyes closed, sometimes your eyeballs can feel restless. If that's the case, focus on the spot that's right between your eyes. Giving them something to aim at should put them at ease.

Don't fight stray thoughts—send them sailing instead. Shutting out every thought is impossible, but when anything floats into your head, don't try to ignore it. Instead, try picturing that thought as a balloon or a sailboat, then watch it drift out of range in your mind.

Need a Nap?

Make the temperature just right. You don't want a spot that's either too warm or too cold. Choosing a dark, comfortable place that falls right in between, temperature-wise, will make you likely to nod much faster and get more from your nap.

Know the limits. Even though everyone is different, most experts agree that keeping a nap between ten and thirty minutes is best. Any longer and you risk falling into a deeper sleep that could cause grogginess and could affect how well you sleep at night.

Stick with naps in the afternoon. The best time for a nap is midafternoon between one and three p.m. The reason? That's when your body usually experiences a natural dip in temperature, which is why some people experience post-lunch sleepiness or a lower level of alertness.

Ready to Reap More from Your Sleep?

Access your zzz needs. You don't need some high-tech life tracker to know if you're not getting enough sleep. Just listen to your body's warning signs. Yawning constantly, having difficulty concentrating or remembering facts, and/or being unexpectedly irritable can all be symptoms of needing more shut-eye.

Stick to the same slumber schedule. Always try to go to bed and get up at the same time every day. Sleeping in on the weekend or on days off may feel deliciously decadent, but it can sometimes disrupt your sleep cycle when you're back on the clock.

Invest in your rest. Look around your bedroom to see if there's anything you could upgrade or change to improve how you spend your nights. From new blinds that let in less light to new sheets that may be more comfy, the changes you make could influence how often your sleep gets disrupted and how long you stay in a deeper, more productive doze.

Dial things back before packing it in. Unwind your mind an hour before bedtime by avoiding things that are too stimulating, such as work, a challenging book, an intense phone conversation, or anything that requires a great deal of focus or energy. And while I'm often guilty of this, try to avoid electronics with screens. (Their glow can sometimes suppress the sleep hormone melatonin.)

Sleep only when sleepy. If you find yourself still awake after trying to sleep for twenty minutes, don't fight it. Instead, get up, keep the lights either off or dimmed, and do something boring until you feel sleepy. Just don't turn on your TV, computer, tablet, or smart phone. Exposure to bright light may signal your brain to stay awake. But since you'll probably do it anyway, try not to do any work on those devices. That'll really tax the brain and affect your ability to fall back asleep.

Watch what you eat, drink, or pop in your mouth. Avoiding caffeinated drinks like coffee, tea, and soda for at least six hours before bedtime is a no-brainer. But other things, including chocolate, nicotine, and certain pain relievers (such as Excedrin or Midol) also contain caffeine and should be avoided when possible before bedtime.

Exercise with caution. For some people, exercising or doing some physical activity close to bedtime works great to knock them out. But for others, elevating the heart rate prior to sleep may leave them more alert, which could make falling asleep more of a chore.

Avoid alcohol if you want a sounder sleep. Alcohol may make you feel tired, but it also affects REM sleep—the restorative type of sleep that happens about ninety minutes after you're out. Drinking too much can make whatever REM you are getting much less effective.

Taper off your sips. If you find yourself waking up at least once a night to use the bathroom, watch how much water you're drinking an hour or two before bedtime. Even if each trip takes only a few minutes, you could end up disrupting the time your body stays in deeper, more restorative sleep.

The "So You Know" Science

Taking five-minute breaks—whether you work as a desk jockey, perform heavy labor, or fall anywhere in between—has multiple benefits beyond helping you unwind, from increasing your concentration, alertness, and work speed to reducing your risk of soreness, musculoskeletal disorders, eyestrain, and even on-the-job accidents. Short breaks have even been linked to having a smaller waistline, lower body mass index (BMI), and lower triglyceride levels, according to the Centers for Disease Control and Prevention.[1]

Perform a 20-Minute Workout 3X a Week

SIMPLY PUT . . . I want you to do some form of a 20-minute full-body strength-training workout three times a week. As part of following this Change, you'll stop doing Change #5 (doing 50 reps of two different exercises), but you'll continue to walk 10,000 steps each day.

An actual conversation with my parents recently

ME: I put together a twenty-minute beginner workout for you two today.

DAD: I walked down the driveway to get the mail this morning and it took about five minutes so I only need another fifteen, right?

MOM: Well, if he's only doing fifteen, then so am I. I brought that bag of clothes down from the attic, and that was heavy!

ME: Guys, guys!! "Existing" doesn't count as exercise. Plus, this is a head-to-toe cardio and strength-training workout.

DAD: Strength training??? Your mother and I don't want to bulk up.

I've had this same conversation with my parents half a dozen times. And while it always makes me laugh, it also frustrates me to no end. I can spend three hundred pages explaining the virtues of strength training, the importance of exercising, and the likelihood of bulking up from it (slim to zilch), but until you're ready to take this next step, I can't do much. That's why we waited for you to get used to nine other Changes before your first workout. We're easing into this so you understand it, feel comfortable with it (as comfortable as sweat can feel), and get excited about it. So let's do this.

When it comes to building lean muscle tissue, boosting your metabolism, and burning more calories and overall body fat in the shortest amount of time, it takes a high-intensity, full-body plan that stimulates as many muscle fibers as possible. Since sticking with Change #5, you've been preparing your muscles for just such a routine.

And before you come up with an excuse as to why you can't start today—or any day—I've made every workout in this book excuse-proof, so they can be done anywhere, anytime, with any amount of space or budget.

Don't have any weights? Great! You won't need a lick of equipment or a gym membership to pull off this program.

Don't have much space? Fine. All you need (at most) is a 6 × 6 foot area to exercise in.

Don't have tons of time? Really? You don't have twenty minutes? That's nothing, and I promise, you'll accomplish more in twenty than most people manage to do working out for an hour.

My whole philosophy when it comes to strength training is to combine cardiovascular exercise and resistance training, along with moves that challenge your core, balance, and flexibility, in each workout. You're already walking 10k steps a day and eating better, so let's maximize the time you spend working out so you're not wasting a minute of time. My goal is to try and utilize as many muscle groups as possible in as few moves as possible, using little bursts of exercises (or mini-circuits) that force you to push through an entire set before resting.

Moving from one exercise to the next with no rest in between will elevate your heart rate throughout the entire workout in the exact same way cardiovascular exercise does, letting you achieve the same fat-burning results. But better still—the less time you rest between exercises, the more you'll rev up your metabolism and the longer it will stay that way after you exercise.

The Game Plan: This 20-minute full-body workout is composed of five quick circuits, each one a combination of several exercises that you'll do back-to-back with no rest in between. After each mini-circuit, you'll rest for sixty to ninety seconds, then move on to the next mini-circuit until you finish all five mini-circuits.

Depending on your skill and comfort level, you can choose to do the workout once through or try to get through it twice for a full 40-minute workout. Just like Change #5, there are no tips, there are no tricks—only a few rules I need you to stick with to get the most from the workout:

1. **Before every workout, do a quick five-minute warm-up.** It takes only a few minutes of light exercise at a low intensity to increase blood flow to your muscles and joints to make them looser, more pliable, and prepared for what's ahead.

2. **Any low-intensity activity will work**—jogging in place, walking in place while pumping your arms back and forth, casually skipping rope (even pretending to skip will work), or if you have access to a piece of stationary equipment, exercising at a low level or gear.

3. **Just remember the "five for five" rule of thumb.** Once you've warmed up for five minutes, you have up to five minutes to start the workout. After that, blood can quickly get shuttled away from your muscles, so don't let yourself be distracted.

4. **Take one day off between sessions.** No matter how hard you push your muscles, you'll still need a full forty-eight hours' recovery time to give them enough time to rest and rebuild between workouts.

5. **Work out in the morning if possible.** If you've ever heard that working out in the morning burns more body fat, there's something to that theory. That's because when you wake up, your body's glycogen reserve—the stored carbohydrates it uses for energy—are depleted. This can cause your body to use a greater percentage of stored fat for energy when you work out.

My personal opinion: Get up, do it in the morning, get it over with, and it will be done for the day. If you leave it dangling at the bottom of your to-do list, it's very easy to cancel.

But if you only have time to work out at night, then go for it. Find your peak time to push yourself, the time of day when you have the most energy, the most time, and the most focus. Do it when you *can* do it, when you *want* to do it, and when you *feel good* about doing it.

6. **If you can exercise on an empty stomach, that's fine**—so long as it doesn't keep you from giving it your all every time. Just know that as you begin performing longer workouts later on in the book, I'll be insisting that you have a little something before every workout.

7. **Don't let your body trick you.** Anytime you're eager to achieve faster results, you're more likely to cheat—whether you're conscious of it or not. That might mean altering your posture to make some of the moves in this workout less difficult to perform. It's just your body's way of trying to make it easier for itself.

But not using proper form will only cheat certain muscles out of a great workout while placing unnecessary stress on other parts of your body. So pay attention as you go. If something that used to feel like a challenge suddenly feels much less demanding, you might be making adjustments to make the exercise easier to do.

THE WORKOUT

Mini-Circuit #1

(Do this circuit once)

- 20 apple pickers
- 20 jogs in place
- 16 apple pickers
- 16 jogs in place
- 12 apple pickers
- 12 jogs in place
- 8 apple pickers
- 8 jogs in place
- 4 apple pickers
- 4 jogs in place

Mini-Circuit #2

(Do this circuit 2 times in a row)

- 50 shoulder circles (forward)
- 10 jumping jacks
- 50 shoulder circles (backward)
- 10 jumping jacks
- 100 reverse claps
- 10 jumping jacks
- 50 reverse claps
- 10 jumping jacks

Mini-Circuit #3

(Do this circuit 3 times in a row)

- 50 hip raises
- 15 toy soldiers

Mini-Circuit #4

(Do this circuit 2 times in a row)

- 20 upper cuts
- 20 quad drops
- 20 wide-leg shuffles in place

Mini-Circuit #5

- 10 front kicks (left leg, right leg = 1 rep), immediately followed by 10 squats
- 9 front kicks (each leg), immediately followed by 9 squats
- 8 front kicks (each leg), immediately followed by 8 squats
- 7 front kicks (each leg), immediately followed by 7 squats
- 6 front kicks (each leg), immediately followed by 6 squats
- 5 front kicks (each leg), immediately followed by 5 squats
- 4 front kicks (each leg), immediately followed by 4 squats
- 3 front kicks (each leg), immediately followed by 3 squats
- 2 front kicks (each leg), immediately followed by 2 squats
- 1 front kick (each leg), immediately followed by 1 squat

THE EXERCISES

Apple Pickers (see page 30)

Jogs in Place

THE MOTION: Stand straight and begin running in place at a pace that has your feet touching the floor at about 60 steps a minute. As you go, swing your arms back and forth (elbows bent at a 90-degree angle) and keep your head up—don't look down at your feet.

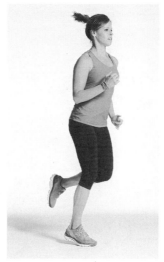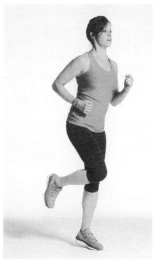

Shoulder Circles (Forward and Backward)

SETUP: Stand straight with your feet together and your arms extended straight out from your sides, palms facing out—you should look like the letter T.

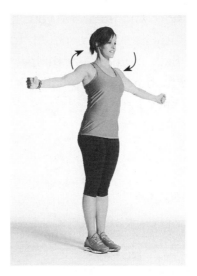

THE MOTION (FORWARD): Keeping your arms straight, make small clockwise circles with your arms. One small circle equals 1 rep.

THE MOTION (BACKWARD): Keeping your arms straight, make small counterclockwise circles with your arms. One small circle equals 1 rep.

Jumping Jacks

SETUP: Stand straight with your arms at your sides and your feet and legs together.

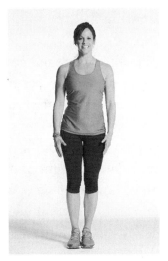

THE MOTION: Quickly sweep your arms out from your sides and up above your head as you simultaneously jump high enough to spread your feet wider than shoulder-width apart. Quickly reverse the motion by hopping back into the setup position. (That's 1 rep.)

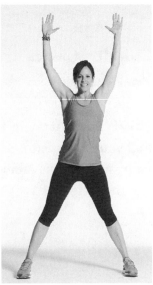

Reverse Claps

SETUP: Stand straight with your arms extended behind you, palms facing each other.

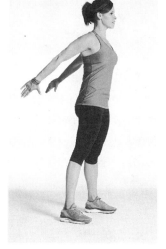

THE MOTION: Keeping your arms straight (or as straight as possible because of the angle), quickly move your arms in and out toward each other as if you were applauding, but don't let your hands touch each other. Instead, try to get them as close as possible without touching. Bringing your arms in and pulling them out equals 1 rep.

Note: The higher you can raise your arms as you go, the more you'll work the back of your arms—but don't hunch over or look down.

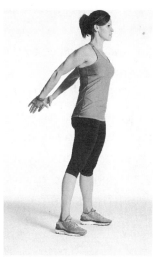

Hip Raises (see page 32)

Supine Finger-to-Toe Touches

SETUP: Lie flat on your back on a mat (or carpeted floor) with your arms extended out from your sides and your feet wider than shoulder-width apart.

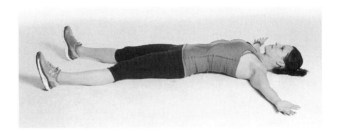

THE MOTION: Slowly raise your right leg and reach your left hand to touch your toes (or reach as close to your toes as you can). Your left shoulder should come up off the floor as you curl up. Lower yourself back down to the floor and repeat, this time by touching your right hand to your left foot. (That's 1 rep.)

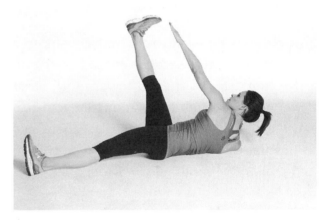

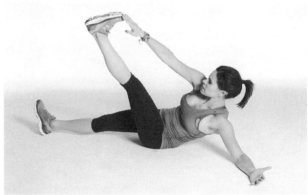

Upper Cuts

SETUP: Stand with your feet wider than shoulder-width apart and knees slightly bent. Bring your fists up by your chin, palms facing in toward your face, elbows pointing down.

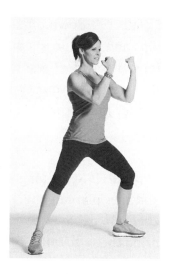

THE MOTION: Keeping your fists in close to your body, quickly punch your right fist straight up directly in front of your face as you simultaneously pull your left fist down. Reverse the motion by quickly punching your left fist straight up directly in front of your face as you simultaneously pull your right fist down. (That's 1 rep.)

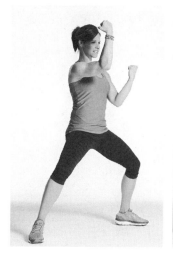 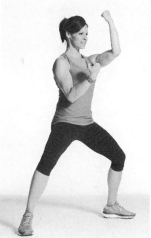

Quad Drops

SETUP: Get down on all fours so that your knees are directly under your hips and your wrists directly under your shoulders. Instead of letting the tops of your feet rest on the floor, curl your toes toward your knees so the bottom of your toes is touching the floor. Finally, raise your knees up so they are suspended off the floor an inch or two.

THE MOTION: Keeping your hands flat and toes planted, quickly raise your knees up off the floor about a foot, then bring them down to the floor without letting them touch down. (That's 1 rep.) Continue to bounce your knees up and down without letting them touch the floor.

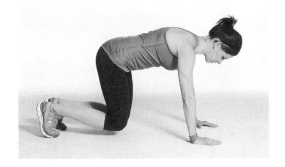

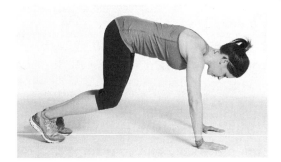

Wide-Leg Shuffles

SETUP: Stand straight with your feet wider than shoulder-width apart, toes angled slightly outward. Extend your arms in front of you, palms pressed firmly together.

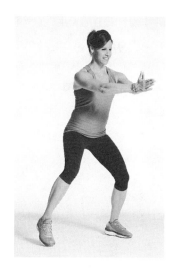

THE MOTION: Keeping your arms extended and palms pressed, raise your heels off the floor (so that you're balanced only on your toes and the balls of your feet) and quickly shift your weight from foot to foot as fast as possible. Imagine the floor is red hot—so hot that you have to keep your feet from touching the floor for more than a split second. Shifting your weight from your left foot to your right, then from your right foot to your left, counts as 1 rep.

Note: Don't look down at your feet, but focus on keeping your toes angled slightly out as you go.

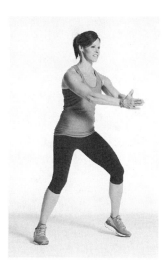

Front Kicks

SETUP: Stand with your feet shoulder-width apart. Bring your fists up by your chin, palms facing each other, with your elbows pointing down.

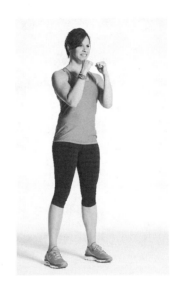

THE MOTION: In one motion, shift your weight to your left foot as you raise your right knee straight up in front of you, then extend your foot forward. Draw your right foot back in, then lower your right leg back to the setup position. Repeat the move with your left leg. (That's 1 rep.)

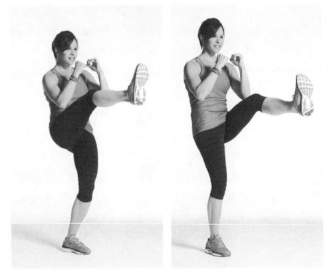

Note: If you're having problems staying balanced, stand with your knees slightly bent and feet shoulder-width apart in a staggered stance. (That means one foot should be a small step in front of the other.) Kick out whichever leg is forward, then quickly switch positions to put the opposite leg forward, then kick again using the opposite leg. Continue to quickly switch positions throughout the set.

Squats (see page 36)

The "So You Know" Science

I'm not the only one who preaches strength training. In fact, there are actual recommendations on the quantity and quality of exercise you should be getting. According to the American College of Sports Medicine, the average adult should train each major muscle group two or three days each week, waiting at least forty-eight hours between strength-training sessions.

That type of training doesn't have to mean lifting weights. Strength training is by definition any exercise that forces your muscles to contract under some form of resistance. That resistance can come from almost anyplace: dumbbells, a barbell, an exercise machine, a stretch cord, or even your own bodyweight (which is the only thing you'll need for every routine in my book).

#11
Consider Your Wardrobe Carefully

SIMPLY PUT . . . Dress to your strength. Whenever you choose an outfit for the day or for the gym or for a big event, pick the things that will help you feel empowered.

I've never been into fashion. I don't gravitate toward labels. I don't wear what's trendy. And I certainly don't wear anything uncomfortable.

I know what you're thinking . . . Who would wear anything uncomfortable? Well, welcome to the wonderful world of television. Those crazy heels and sleeveless dresses in the dead of winter? Uncomfortable. I like what I like and I often stay under the radar on the clothing spectrum.

It's easy to look back and pinpoint exactly when my indifference toward clothing came about. It was 1989, I had just moved to the United States from the Caribbean, where I had lived for fourteen years—and I was about to start high school. Woo-hoo!!! High school as the new kid in class! For some reason, that sounded awesome, thanks in part to living in Haiti. I never saw an *Afterschool Special*, so I knew nothing about high school hardships.

The weekend before school started, my mom took me to a discount store and bought me a few outfits for my first week in ninth grade. I laid out all the new clothes on my bed and picked out what I deemed would be my first-day-of-high-school **Power Outfit**: red pants, a white button-down short-sleeved top with some colorful coconut trees stamped everywhere, and loafers (I'll pause for a moment so you can fully take that in).

Looking back, I'm not surprised I was the laughingstock of my freshman class. And while I chuckle about it now, it was heartbreaking back then. No matter what I wore or how hard I tried to fit in, my wardrobe kept me out and I never quite caught up. I was always much more productive (and happy) dressing down comfortably than dressing up uncomfortably.

Granted, being on television forced me to adjust my fashion focus a little bit. But when I'm not on TV, I'm out of my fancy dress and heels and back to dressing for strength and comfort. Jeans, a soft T-shirt, a worn-in sweater, and a pair of boots—Boom, I'm done! And while much of the world enjoys Fashion Week, a good high-end shoe sale, or when Oscar goers are asked who they're wearing on the red carpet, I tune out.

I tune most fashion out, but I still recognize that I am better when I feel better...and I feel better when I dress strong. Whether its color, style, or fit, I dress the way I want to feel. For me, I know I deliver a better speech when I'm wearing a black power dress. I know I'll feel happier and more confident on a summer weekend when I'm wearing flip-flops. And when I exercise, while it's still not about what brands I'm wearing, I dress the part.

For me, I know that I personally work out harder and more effectively when I'm wearing my favorite gym colors, which are gray and either yellow or orange. So why does it matter what I wear to the gym? I don't want to hide my body under baggy clothes because that prevents me from being accountable. Wearing tight clothes or showing a little skin means that if there's any part of me that needs to be addressed, it's there to mock (and motivate) me when I walk in front of every mirror.

But even though you and I may be different, the concept of picking outfits that either inspire you to be more active or remind you what you need to work on is a tactic anyone can use. And I'm not just talking about what you wear to exercise. I'm talking about your entire wardrobe—every last piece of attire folded in your dresser and hanging in your closet.

I may not love fashion, but that doesn't mean I don't think about what I'm wearing every day. Believe it or not, what you wear can go a long way toward keeping your food in check and burning calories all day long.

Tips and Tricks

For me, if I don't like what I see in the mirror, I will do something about it. But maybe for you, seeing your flaws reflected back leaves you feeling self-conscious and more likely to race through your workouts or skip them altogether. No matter what your personality (or style!) may be, these apparel pointers will still let you get more from the Changes you've already triumphed over and the ones you'll soon be tackling.

With Your Workout Clothes

Find your power colors. Now you know mine, but I didn't know them right away. It was a matter of trial and error. Try to mix up what you wear each time and see if you notice any difference in your performance. Best bet: Make sure to take it a step further and wear colors you normally never wear—you may be surprised at what fires you up when it's time to sweat.

Don't have a power color? If seeing your problem areas drives you, try wearing bright colors that accentuate your "need to work on" parts and dark colors to hide your "right on track" spots. If seeing your problem areas keeps you from putting in as much effort, just do the exact opposite.

Keep it plain if you can't plan. If coordinating clothes isn't your thing, I'd rather you keep things as simple as possible than skip a workout. Instead, when it comes to bottoms, stick with black, white, or gray—all three pretty much go with anything, so whatever you grab to wear up top should match in a pinch.

Leave it lean if weighing less is your goal. Even if you hate pointing out your problem spots, stick with slimmer-fitting clothes that hug your frame instead of hiding it. Looser clothing not only makes you look heavier, but it may prevent you from checking your posture as you exercise. The more you can see your silhouette, the less often you'll exercise incorrectly.

If you can't move in it, make another choice. Anything you wear should always fit comfortably. If you love Lycra or spandex, I'm not going to stop you. But if it's tight anyplace on your body that bends—waist, shoulders, knees, elbows, wrists, ankles, and even your neck—either stretch it out or switch it out to give yourself more freedom.

Never skimp on your shoes. It's not hype. There actually is a difference among walking, running, and cross-trainer shoes in terms of their support, padding, breathability, and structure. Investing in one pair of walking shoes for your 10,000 steps and a pair of cross-trainers for your workouts can help reduce your risk of injury and improve your performance.

Just remember when to replace them! Toss your walking/running shoes for a pair of new ones every three to five hundred miles. Your cross-trainers should be good for about a year before you need a new pair, so long as you're only wearing them when you exercise.

...And the Rest of Your Wardrobe

Think fitted over forgiving. Ample room and elastic waistbands are not your friends, because they let you get away with ignoring your body, along with the warning signs that you may be eating too much. Instead, stick with non-stretch jeans and clothes with enough room to spare but snug enough to remind you of your goals.

Buy one outfit in your target size. I'm not saying go crazy, but spend a few bucks on something simple—a swimsuit, a cheap but cute dress, whatever—in the size that you *will* be one day. Then hang it behind your bedroom door so it's the first thing you see when you head out for the day and the last thing you see when you go to sleep.

Size down your pj's. There's a reason we love curling up in our jammies. All that extra room makes it way too easy to snack away at night without feeling the pinch around your waistline. Instead, get a pair that's not as forgiving, or if you can't give up the comfort of your old pj's, wear something slightly restrictive underneath that reminds you when your belly's filling up.

If it's baggy, then bag it. As you begin to drop a few pounds, don't just ignore your fat clothes. Toss them in a bag and put them somewhere that's out of sight and inconvenient. The fewer oversized options you have at your disposal, the more likely you'll be to reach for an outfit that's less forgiving.

Size up what you need. It's far from an exact science, but for every five to ten pounds you lose, you typically will drop one size. Each time that happens, buy (or better yet borrow) just a few wardrobe essentials, such as a pair of black pants, one pair of jeans, a fitted blouse, or even a day dress and evening dress, so you have just a few things that fit the new you perfectly during those "in-between" stages.

Bring your belt in a notch. Instead of wearing it to fit (or ever letting it out!), cinch your belt up a hole when you're not sitting down. That tiny bit of constraint can sometimes help keep you more conscious of your eating habits and activity levels throughout the day.

Embrace casual Fridays. The more comfortable you dress during the day, the more active you're likely to be.

The "So You Know" Science

A now-classic study performed at the University of Wisconsin found that wearing casual, comfortable clothing to work (over conventional business attire) actually affects your physical activity level. According to the research, when participants wore jeans, they walked an average of 491 (or 8 percent) more steps and burned an average of 25 more calories a day.[1]

That may not sound like much, but keep in mind that when added up, wearing casual clothing to work every day equals 125 calories a week (or 6,250 calories in a fifty-week year). It's a difference researchers believe could help offset the average annual weight gain of 0.4 to 1.8 pounds that American adults naturally experience as they age.

#12
Covertly Work Your Core Throughout the Day

SIMPLY PUT . . . Imagine how you'd react if someone were about to punch you in the stomach. You'd tighten that midsection and brace yourself for the blow. Do you see how you squeezed your stomach muscles but didn't suck in your gut? That's what I want you to do all the time.

For me, the core is the key to everything.

Building core strength—in other words, having strong abdominal, lower back, and oblique muscles (the ones you hide underneath your love handles)—is key if your goal is getting and staying strong, balanced, and healthy.

Will training these muscles lead to a flatter, leaner midsection? The short answer is yes, but core work doesn't mean sit-ups and crunches. Your core—the major muscles that move, support, and stabilize your spine—affect your strength, endurance, flexibility, motor control, and function. You'd need a lot more than crunches to tackle all that. So to fully work your core, you need to broaden your abdominal horizons.

Your core is your center of gravity, and when it's conditioned, it's what keeps your body in perfect alignment. That means less back pain, better balance and posture, and a major improvement in practically any task you can think of. To put it another way, a strong core can lead to a strong everything else.

So let's get back to the anticipated punch in the gut. By bracing your stomach as if you were going to absorb the blow, you work your core from the inside out. Keeping it contracted all the time can help tighten your midsection—without ever having to step foot in a gym. But it's not that easy.

In the beginning, you'll have to consciously think about it—otherwise you'll forget and let your stomach out. When I first tried this, I considered it a success if I kept my core tight for five straight minutes. After a month, I had worked up to an hour straight. I was constantly reminding myself: Tight core. Tight core. Tight core. At the gym. In the shower. On TV. Keep it tight. Keep it tight!

Today, I no longer think about it. It now takes a conscious effort for me to completely let my stomach out. Both times I was pregnant, I found that subconsciously I was holding my core in. When someone took a picture of me pregnant, I had to remind myself to let my stomach out to show off what my belly looked like.

One time, Bill Murray visited the set to promote a movie he was doing. Somewhere between my attempts to impress him with how many lines I remember from *Caddyshack* (like three...so pathetic), we decided to take a belly-to-belly picture to compare physiques. His golf body and my pregnant body. I'll never forget purposely letting my stomach out to look more pregnant for the picture.

I'm fully expecting that when my children get older, they'll both ask me, "OK, what in the hell *was that* for the first nine months?"

DON'T STOP THERE...

First things first: It's not about sucking your stomach in and holding your breath for fourteen hours. It's about doing what comes naturally to you. If I were to punch you in the gut, you wouldn't just stand there and suck your stomach in. (You'd be the easiest target ever.) No, you would automatically contract all of your core muscles without thinking about it. And that's what I'm asking you to do all day (and eventually all night) long.

Don't overdo it—there's no need to. You still need to function and perform your regular everyday activities, right? All I'm asking you to do is make a muscle, and you'll find a happy medium between that and what you're comfortable walking around doing.

Once you get the hang of doing it, it's about reminding yourself to do it. When I first started out, I had to remind myself every thirty seconds to tighten my core, which quickly turned into every few minutes, then every hour. But within a couple of months, I was doing it all the time without any thought at all.

Eventually, you'll get to that same point. Right now, your stomach may be hanging out and it's a chore to even think about holding it in. But I promise you: Before you finish the thirty Changes, it'll become so second nature to you that the only effort will be inflating it when you want to pretend you're eating for two.

Tips and Tricks

It's your core muscles that decide how powerful and pain-free the rest of your body is, and working them all day long in little ways can add up to a big payoff. Here are some techniques to activate them instantly in a few subtle ways.

Make like a flamingo. Anytime you're standing around in one place, bend one knee slightly and lift your foot at least an inch off the ground (either behind or in front of you) so you're balancing on one leg. Start with thirty seconds on each foot and then increase that to a minute—you'll be engaging your core the entire time. It doesn't matter whether you're pouring a cup of coffee, brushing your teeth, waiting in line to buy another copy of this book for a friend, or standing in an elevator—try it wherever it's safe, feasible, and sometimes inconspicuous.

I say *sometimes* because I used to do it while I was on the air at the *Today* show all the time. Standing on the plaza in the dead of winter, I would lift one foot up and contract all my muscles to stay warm. There I was, dressed up for TV—hair, makeup, and fancy dress—balancing on one six-inch heel on live television. Did I risk kissing the pavement? Every time! But did I get some much needed core work in despite that risk? Absolutely.

Lift and lean. If you find yourself sitting on something stable without a backrest, allowing you to lean (like a bleacher seat or bench, for example), try this: Shimmy your butt to the edge, straighten your legs, raise your feet off the floor, then lean back (keeping your back straight) so that you're balancing your body like a seesaw. Hold for as long as you can, rest, and repeat.

Plank while you lounge. The next time you're lying belly down on the floor (playing a board game with your kids, reading this book, surfing on your tablet, and so forth), use that time to plank. Get yourself in a classic push-up position—legs extended straight behind you, feet wider than shoulder-width apart—then rest on your forearms so that your arms are at 90-degree angles. Your body should form a straight line from your head to your heels. Don't let your midsection sag down or pop up. See page 120 to learn how. Once in plank, hold that pose for as long as possible—the longer you lounge, the better you'll be for it.

Engage behind the engine. Whenever you're stuck riding in a car for a long time, put your hands flat on the roof, then gently press up with your arms as you tighten your midsection. Try it for ten to twenty seconds when you hit a light or are stuck in traffic.

Get a leg up when your butt's down. If you're seated in a sturdy chair (at work, at home, in a restaurant, even at the movies), sit up as straight as possible, tighten your core, then raise one foot six inches off the floor. Hold that pose for as long as you comfortably can, repeat it with the opposite leg, then alternate back and forth.

If you want a tougher challenge, try lifting both feet off the floor at the same time while maintaining perfect posture. I once did this for the entire length of a feature film (not the previews) at the movie theater and spent the next day not only boring my friends to death with every detail of the experiment but with a sore core as well.

The "So You Know" Science

If you're "core-curious," the primary muscles that make up your core aren't just your abs, love handles, and lower back. Yes, your abs (officially known as your rectus abdominis muscle) are responsible for bending your torso forward, your lower back (or erector spinae) raises your torso and lets you bend your torso backward, and your internal and external obliques, the muscles along your sides that help you rotate your torso and bend it from side to side. But the other players that never get any credit include your transverse abdominis (a thin band of muscle that runs across your midsection that compresses your abdomen and draws your belly button toward your spine), and your lumbar multifidi (the tiny muscles that connect your vertebrae to one another and hold your spine stable during movement).

#13

Aim for a 500-Calorie Deficit Every Day

SIMPLY PUT . . . I want you to either eat 500 calories fewer than usual each day or burn an extra 500 calories each day. You can also reach a happy medium by doing a combination of both—eating fewer calories and exercising—until you hit that 500-calorie deficit.

I know.

I know.

That sounds daunting, doesn't it? Five hundred of anything sounds daunting. But 500 actual calories? Think about this though. If you can achieve a 500-calorie deficit every day for a week (either by eating 500 fewer calories a day, burning 500 more calories a day, or a combination of both), you'll lose a pound. Yes, just one in a whole week, because as I told you in Change #3, one pound equals 3,500 calories.

Losing just a pound a week may not sound like much, but it gives you ammunition for those who insist on rushing the process. The next time someone tells you they're going on some crazy diet to lose fifteen pounds for a wedding next week, explain the caloric math to them: To shave fifteen pounds in a week, they'll have to burn 52,500 calories—*fifty-two thousand!!!* Then watch how quickly they readjust that number.

But here's the good news: Because of the changes you've incorporated into your lifestyle since starting this plan, you're probably already creating that 500-calorie deficit. That means that what seems like the hardest Change to make in this book may be the easiest one in the bunch.

According to experts, the best way to create that 500-calorie deficit is by doing a combination of cardiovascular exercise to burn calories, strength training to build lean muscle and boost your metabolism, and modifying your diet. You know, pretty much what you're doing already, now that you're twelve Changes into this program. In fact, just a few of the Changes that are helping you hit well over that 500-calorie mark right now include:

- **Change #3 (Walking 10k steps a day):** This alone can burn roughly **250** calories.
- **Change #4 (No carbs after 6:00 p.m.):** I can't see what you've been eating, but it has to be fewer calories through smarter choices. I'll be conservative and say you're eating about **300** fewer calories every night.
- **Change #6 (Redo how you chew):** By chewing your food at least twenty times, you're most likely doubling the number of chews you used to take before starting this program. If that's the case, you're eating (on average) **112** fewer calories **per meal** (or 15 percent less food) according to research published in the *Journal of the Academy of Nutrition and Dietetics.*[1]
- **Change #10: (Adding a 20-minute workout three times a week):** Depending on how much you weigh, you're burning anywhere from **150** to **250** additional calories each day you perform this high-intensity routine.

DON'T STOP THERE...

As a result of the Changes you've already mastered—and the Changes you're about to experience—you're going to continue to reach that 500-calorie deficit and lose weight as you build lean muscle. But eventually, depending on how much weight you have to lose, you may hit a point where your weight loss results may peak.

That's when making a few tweaks to either your exercise or eating plan can keep your weight loss efforts moving along.

If You Choose Exercise...

There are obviously certain activities that burn more calories than others—running, hill sprinting, swimming, stair climbing, strength training, cross-country skiing, and skipping rope. But when people ask me what is the "best" exercise they should do to burn calories, my answer is always the same: whatever you love to do. Because if you love doing it, you'll *keep* doing it, and if you *keep* doing it, you'll burn those calories right off.

So if you love to swim, swim. Love heading out on your bike? Then hop on a bike and go. Big fan of hitting a step class when the mood strikes? Then step away. How you choose to get your heart pumping is up to you, so long as it gets your heart rate up for the length of time you're doing it (and occasionally mix it up).

No matter what you pick, here's how many extra calories you'll burn in just ten minutes (based on a 140-pound person):

- Aerobics, general: **63** calories
- Aerobics, high-impact: **74** calories
- Aerobics, low-impact: **53** calories
- Backpacking: **74** calories
- Basketball (just shooting baskets): **48** calories
- Bicycling at a light pace (10 to 11.9 mph): **64** calories
- Bicycling at a moderate pace (12 to 13.9 mph): **84** calories
- Bicycling at a vigorous pace (14 to 15.9 mph): **106** calories
- Dancing (general): **48** calories
- Running (5 mph, or a 12-minute mile): **84** calories
- Running (6 mph, or a 10-minute mile): **106** calories
- Running (7 mph, or a 8.5-minute mile): **121** calories
- Running (8 mph, or a 7.5-minute mile): **143** calories
- Running (9 mph, or a 6.5-minute mile): **159** calories
- Running up stairs: **159** calories
- Skipping rope (slow pace): **84** calories

- Skipping rope (moderate pace): **106** calories
- Skipping rope (rapid pace): **127** calories
- Swimming laps (light to moderate effort): **97** calories
- Swimming laps (fast to vigorous effort): **121** calories

If You Choose Diet...

Most of the day, we are creatures of habit. Even though you've been adjusting what, when, and how you eat through the Changes in this book, odds are, you're probably still eating many of the foods you've always eaten.

Maybe it's that large coffee and whole bagel you usually have for breakfast. Or that special sandwich you buy every Tuesday. Whatever it is, I won't be asking you to count calories. Instead, I'm just going to suggest a few tricks that can help you dial them back even further. Stick with some of the following tips, and when combined with the calorie-reducing Changes you're already making, I guarantee you'll be secretly stripping calories from your diet and creating a 500-calorie deficit without making any major sacrifices—or needing to add them up.

Just a few subtle suggestions:

Eat one less bite at every meal. Many say you could save around 75 calories a day using this trick—so long as you don't make up that missing bite by sneaking in an unscheduled snack later.

Chill, skim, reheat, then eat. You can reduce the fat from many foods (from anything fried to stews and soups) by not eating them on the same day that you cook them. Instead, let them cool in the fridge overnight after cooking them. The next day, just skim off the fat, heat the food back up, and the same meal now has fewer calories.

Make certain meals in reverse. Instead of topping your cereal or ice cream with a few berries or slices of fruit, put the fruit into your bowl first, and then add the rest. You'll end up adding in more fruit and leaving less room for everything else.

Add some volume to your cheese. Instead of adding a slice of cheese to whatever you're eating, shave or grate the cheese on top. When grated, it takes up roughly twice the volume, so you'll end up eating half the amount without noticing the difference.

Put more thought into your toppings. Replace your butter, sour cream, or dressing with salsa, lemon juice, a fruit spread, low-fat or nonfat Greek yogurt, or just use half to one-fourth of what you normally use.

If it's an effort to spread, skip it. If you can't live without your butter or cream cheese, *stick with whipped or softer versions rather than the solid or hard variety.* Hard-packed butter can have 20-plus more calories per tablespoon (and hard-packed cream cheese has about 30 more calories per ounce).

Eat the same meats, but cook them differently. If a food you usually enjoy is something fried or sautéed, bake or broil it instead. If you usually eat something that's baked or broiled, then try having it steamed or smoked.

Choose the next healthiest cut. For beef and pork, opt for less fatty cuts. Anything with the word *rib* in it (rib eye or prime rib, for example) is generally higher in fat. Instead, switch to a cut of meat that either ends in *-loin* (such as top loin, tenderloin, or sirloin) or has the word *round* in it (round steak, top or bottom round, for example).

The "So You Know" Science

The average person burns about 65 to 70 percent of their total daily calories to maintain their body's essential life functions. In other words, your body actually blasts through two-thirds of the calories you eat each day just to keep you upright and alive. (It's like getting 800 free points for simply writing your name down on the SAT test!!)

On top of that, your body spends another 10 percent of the calories you eat just consuming, digesting, and metabolizing your food (otherwise known as the "thermic effect of feeding"). So for every 100 calories you eat, your body has to spend about 10 calories just to process that food.

Surprisingly, your body uses only about 20 to 25 percent of the calories you eat to pull off physical activity (more if you're extremely active, and much less if you're sedentary). And even then, your body burns a few extra calories as a bonus after you've finished an activity and boosted its metabolism. For every 100 calories you burn doing something physical (exercise, sports, chores, etc.), your body burns an additional 15 calories (give or take) afterward.

CHANGE

#14
Reward Yourself

SIMPLY PUT . . . Congratulate yourself on a successful week with a little non-food-based pampering. Come up with a few different ways to treat yourself, then pick one for every additional week you stick with the Changes moving forward.

Look, change is tough, no matter how strong-willed you are. There will be days where it takes absolutely everything out of you. I remember those days vividly when I was trying to drop my baby weight. Those were the days when I needed a little pat on the back. But besides my parents and maybe a houseplant, who was really going to sit there and congratulate me for every pound lost? (*Looks around the room. Silence.*)

Exactly.

So I decided to congratulate myself with my own little incentive program. For every week of success, a small non-food "me" gift. A massage (the ultimate me time), a new pair of sneakers (my favorite fashion splurge), a guitar lesson (I would need to string together a hundred successful weeks in a row to be able to actually play some good songs, but I digress).

As it turned out, pampering myself with little things here and there actually worked. Whether you're doing this program as a 30-day plan or moving along at your own clip, you're about halfway through—and that's fantastic. So think about this: No matter where you are along this journey, you're still light-years ahead of most everyone else (who keep promising to start next Monday), and it's time to pat yourself on the back.

DON'T STOP THERE...

If incentivized motivation works for you, then you'll love this chapter. Again, my rule of thumb is to treat yourself at the end of every week to remind you of the work you put in. But that doesn't mean you can't create a system that's even more motivational for you. Depending on your means, creativity, time, and how effective you find this Change to be, there are a number of ways you could take this:

• You could give yourself a bonus reward at the end of each month, so you look beyond the day-to-day, week-to-week journey we're taking together. (I find that just crossing successful days off on a calendar gives me a feeling of accomplishment at the end of the month.)

• You could strike a deal with your partner that for every day you stay true to all your Changes, you earn ten to fifteen minutes of me time, so at week's end, your partner handles the kids and you get to spend those accrued minutes getting a well-deserved break. (This one always seems to work *in theory.*)

• Instead of rewarding yourself at the same time of the same day every week, enjoy it at your lowest point. Save your reward for whichever day proves to be the most difficult, like dodging all the bad food at your office's midweek meeting or managing to finish all your 10,000 steps on a day when you were stuck behind a desk or were traveling. You'll be giving yourself a bonus for staying true to your Changes when life tries to blow you off course.

Wait...One Last Thing

Even though this reward is *non-food based*, some still feel like they deserve a cheat meal every week. I obviously can't stop that from happening, but what I can do is point out the following:

If you wanted to kick smoking and managed to go a week without a cigarette, would you reward yourself with a cigarette? If you were trying to quit drinking and stopped cold turkey for a whole seven days, would you pat yourself on the back by pouring a drink? Does that make sense to you?

I know comparing smoking and drinking to watching your diet may be like comparing apples to oatmeal. But for some people with a health-compromising weight issue, it can be equally serious. And even if that's not you, does it make any sense to reward yourself by overeating some of the foods that made you into the person you're trying to change in the first place?

I can't stop you from indulging in a sweet, salty, and carby cheat meal, but I can suggest a couple of things to try in its place:

1. **Take your new self out for a test spin.** Do something at the end of the week that used to require more effort or that you couldn't do until now. Maybe it's 50 jumping jacks in a row, or walking up a few flights of steps without being winded, or trying on a pair of pants that used to require the top button be left undone. Whatever it is, big or small, enjoy it. Then ask yourself if the food you're tempted to eat is worth as much as the pride you feel at that moment. (It's not. It never is.)

2. If you're still set on a big meal—**treat yourself to a better meal,** something that won't reverse your success but feels just as indulgent. After a particularly tough but successful week, I'll forgo the plain old grilled fish and instead indulge in lobster.

3. **Make it a real meal, not a snack fest.** It's too easy to lose yourself in a big bag of…well…of junk. Grabbing small handfuls of pretzels, chips, and whatever processed junk you may cheat with may feel like a smarter option, but most people end up eating more in the long run than they would if they had just had one large meal. So stick your snacking hands in your pocket, send me an invite, and let's grab an actual meal!

Tips and Tricks

We're all different, and only you know what's going to feel like a real reward at the end of each week. But if you need some inspiration...

Pick something that boosts your progress. There are plenty of rewards that can actually help you further your fitness goals, such as a personal training session, a new workout top, a piece of exercise equipment, a better water bottle, or even just a new song to listen to when you're walking. (Sometimes, on days when I'm not particularly motivated, all it takes is a new playlist on my iPod to get me in a workout mood.)

Invest in something that accentuates the new you. You're already changing yourself from the inside out, so think of rewards that can spotlight or add to what you've already achieved. A new hairstyle or color, a facial, a manicure/pedicure, etc.

Make it an event to remember. Instead of buying some "thing" for yourself, use it as an excuse to have an experience instead. Treat yourself to a movie or concert, or a sports or theatrical event you've been dying to see.

Choose something that may help you grow. If there's a skill or activity you've always wanted to try, then buy yourself a paid session. It should be something you've put on hold for whatever reason, because you deserve it. A few bucket-list suggestions:

- Learning how to golf, snowboard, or rock climb (Mom, stick to golf please!)
- Taking a drawing, painting, or pottery class
- Learning another language
- Trying a photography or cooking course
- Playing an instrument you've always wanted to try

Make it something that soothes. Whether it's a bubble bath, a spa day, downloading your favorite show, or just making time for a nice long nap without anyone bothering you, give yourself the time to do something that you usually feel guilty doing. Having it be attached to something you should be proud of will take away some of that guilt—trust me.

Give yourself the night—or day—off. If you have someone who's willing, make a deal that for every week you succeed, they have to relieve you of a specific job that's normally your responsibility. For example:

- Getting a break from cooking for a night—or two
- Letting someone else take the garbage out and clean during the week. (Good luck with this one, but it's worth a try.)
- Not having to give the kids a bath or help them do their homework

Not creative? Remember, cash is king. If you don't feel like drumming up any rewards, then give yourself a cash bonus at the end of each week instead. Whether you save it or spend it, just remind yourself that you've earned it.

#15

Prepare Your Meals and Workouts for the Day/Week

(Before you shout "Impossible"...keep reading!)

SIMPLY PUT... Figure out what you want to eat for the next seven days (breakfast, lunch, dinner, and snacks), then take an evening to prepare as many meals as possible. The same planning goes for your workouts and 10,000 steps—grab a calendar and pencil in exactly when and where you plan on fitting in time to exercise/walk.

Look, I'm a work in progress. We are *all* works in progress.

As such, I'm the first to admit that the whole food thing is not easy for me. I don't know how to cook, I absolutely love to eat, and I generally gravitate toward the exact same things every week for breakfast, lunch, and snacks. As for dinner, well, let's just say it's always potluck.

It's easy to blame bad choices on not having enough time to think about what you're going to eat. So here's a novel concept: Think about what you're going to eat—*before* you eat! If you can do that (stocking your house with the things you need, pre-cooking and preparing all of your meals and snacks), it does more than just save time. It causes you to naturally make smarter food choices without trying that hard.

The same prep goes for your workouts. For me, if I have to get up early to exercise, I will grab everything I need—shorts, T-shirt, sports bra, a pair of socks, cover-up, long-sleeved shirt, shoes, earphones, you name it—and place it all down on a table before I go to bed. So when I wake up, I just go down the line, throw it all on in under five minutes, and I'm out the door. The minute I have to search for a clean sports bra or my iPod or the other sock, I'm in trouble. Why? I have the attention span of a lightly scented Eucalyptus candle. The minute I lose focus, I'm off to something else. So don't let yourself lose focus first thing in the morning.

And as you might imagine, it's not just about organizing your clothes. Organizing your workouts is essential too. I have a big desk calendar on the back of my bedroom door. Every day I work out, I pen a little *W* on it for *workout*. Every day I eat well, I pen a little *F* for *food*. The rest of the calendar square is used for writing down my workouts (what I'm doing, where and when). So start writing down your workouts, because what that will do is turn them into an assignment, as opposed to something you need to find a moment to squeeze in.

DON'T STOP THERE...

An actual conversation with my dad

ME: Hey, Dad, what are you up to?

DAD: Just watching the game.

ME: What are you eating?

DAD: Almonds.

ME: Um, you were eating almonds when I called you two hours ago.

DAD: Yeah, I just finished the bag.

ME: Dad, that's like 45,000 calories!!!

DAD: But they're so light, how could they be fattening?

ME: I don't even know what that means. From now on, fill up an Altoids tin of almonds and that's all the almonds you're allowed to eat!

DAD: You mean for breakfast?

ME: *For the whole day!!!!*

If I haven't stressed it enough, I'll say it again: I don't want you to count calories. And one more time for good measure: *No calorie counting.*

What I *do* want you to do though is come to terms with what a normal serving size looks like—at least when it comes to the foods you're eating regularly. (And please don't consult my dad for this.)

Once you see what's considered average, it will be easier for you to see what's not. And smaller portions mean fewer calories, without having to add anything up.

There are a few standard ways to eyeball certain foods without needing a dietician on call or any nutrition app to tell you the score. For example:

- A three-ounce serving of cooked (not raw) chicken, fish, or meat is about the size of a deck of cards (or about the size of a woman's palm).
- A one-cup serving of pasta or rice (cooked) is about the size of a tennis ball (or a normal scoop of ice cream).
- A one-ounce serving of nuts, pretzels, or chips is roughly one handful.
- A one-ounce serving of cheese is around the size of two pairs of dice.
- A normal single serving of fruit or vegetables is the size of a tennis ball.
- A single serving of green salad is about the size of an open-cupped hand.
- A normal-sized baked potato is the size of a baseball.
- A standard serving of cereal is about whatever you can pour into an average-sized coffee cup (or about the size of a baseball).
- A teaspoon-sized serving of fats, oils, or butter is around the size of the tip of your thumb.
- A normal single serving of salad dressing is about the size of your thumb.
- A serving of peanut butter (two tablespoons) is about the size of a Ping-Pong ball.

But here's the thing: I don't know how big your hands are. They could be as small as a credit card or the size of my friend Kaitlyn's, who can palm a watermelon. So come up with something in between that works for you and stick to it.

Like I always tell my parents when they swear they're only eating one serving of nuts and the one serving turns out to be a camp trunk, I always use an Altoids tin to measure out a single serving of nuts, and I've used coffee cups to measure out my cereal. You make do with what's around you.

So try this: For the first couple of times you're preparing food, use a few measuring tools—a measuring cup, teaspoon, tablespoon, and a food scale (if you have one)—to see a normal serving size of the foods you eat. Then ask yourself how big that serving size really is.

Hey, if you think a serving of fish looks more like the size of a checkbook or the sponge in your bathtub instead of a deck of cards, I'm not going to debate you. Create and use your own visual cues, and whatever helps you remember what a normal portion should look like, stick with it.

Trust me—within a few weeks, the serving sizes of everything you typically eat will become ingrained in your brain and you'll always know (without needing any tools) when you're preparing bigger portions than your body really needs.

Tips and Tricks

The plan is simple—plan! But even though you already know what to do, using a few of these tactics can make the most of all your prep work.

Shop for your meals—not for yourself. Buying food without an agenda is like giving your appetite a license to kill. Having a plan and a grocery list makes distractions minimal, so write a list of only the items you need to make your meals for the week ahead and shop for only those items.

Fill your freezer with frozen foods—but not the bad kinds. Instead of messing with all fresh ingredients, take advantage of a few bags of bulk frozen meats, vegetables, and fruits. Frozen foods are often cheaper than fresh, they are already washed, peeled, and cut, and because these foods are processed and frozen immediately, they typically retain more nutrients.

Grab your takeout menus and circle the good stuff. Instead of hoping you'll make a healthy decision during those "high-pressure, low-willpower" moments when ordering in, go through *all* of your takeout menus (on a full stomach) and circle the smartest choice on each menu so you're never caught off guard. Bonus points for grabbing menus from other local restaurants you haven't been to yet—but could find yourself at with friends or coworkers one day—and doing the same as added insurance.

Invest in a cooler. Being able to eat healthy at any time, no matter where you are, can make all the difference. Keeping healthy snacks (such as fruit, nut mixes, protein bars, a can of tuna, packets of almond butter, or whole-grain crackers) in your car, at your office, or in your bag will give you the convenience of having healthier foods close by.

Take your time. Spending a few extra minutes to measure portions and trim away a little excess fat may take more time, but I guarantee you that for every extra minute you spend in your kitchen, you're probably sparing yourself from two or three minutes of exercise. Trust me— It takes less time to prepare a lighter meal or snack than it does to burn off whatever extra calories you might have eaten if you hadn't prepared ahead of time.

Don't let your workout clothes stray far from one another. Invest in a few single-mesh laundry bags (two should be fine). Then as soon as you're through with your workout, toss everything into the bag—shirt, sports bra, shorts, sweats, even your underwear and socks. Cinch it up and throw it in the wash. That way, you'll have everything in one place for the next workout without wasting time scrambling to find things, or worse, not exercising at all.

Pay close attention to what Mr. Roker says. Getting in your 10,000 steps becomes a lot harder when Mother Nature has other plans. Watch the weeklong forecast and prepare for the worst. If the news says "chance of rain" (or anything else that might keep you indoors), assume that the chance will be 100 percent and figure out what indoor activities you can do to help hit that 10k goal. And if it said rain but you got sun, I'm giving you carte blanche to blame Al.

Prepare for a week, but think ahead for three more. Look on your calendar to see if there are any events, holidays, loosely planned meetings, dates, anything that could sideline your efforts down the road, then make sure you have a contingency plan.

Today show Tested

The first time I heard about meal preps was on the set of the *Today* show. I was getting ready to go on air with a story when I overheard nutritionist (and friend) Joy Bauer explaining to someone how easy it is for her to eat well because she prepares all her meals for the week on Sunday night.

Wait, what did she say? She cooks for a week in one night? One night?? *All her meals?* I honestly thought it was the start of a joke. I literally remember smiling as I walked past her and onto the set. "What a nut job," I thought. (I can say that because Joy and I are good friends who exchange the term of not-so-much endearment with each other often.) But she wasn't kidding!

Later that morning, I was in my office when my former colleague (and friend) Erica Hill popped in. She had been up late the night before—making all her dinners for the week.

"Hold on," I said. "Do you live with Joy Bauer??"

Turns out, Erica does this as well and uses it as a way to battle the three things she has working against her during the week: time, culinary creativity, and willpower.

So after inviting myself over to her place for dinner for 364 days next year (I didn't want to be greedy), I decided to quietly give this new approach to food a try on a Sunday night. I used the word *try* because, unlike Joy and Erica, who are both fantastic cooks, I am not. I'm barely a preparer. I'm not even really a gatherer. I tend to eat either what's in front of me or what's in front of others.

Apparently, I was right about dinner (I'll spare you the details). I'm not great at it, but I found that breakfast, lunch, and snacks were quite doable. Boiling all my hard-boiled eggs in one night helped me get my protein in every morning during the week. I also cut up fruits and vegetables to bring to work as snacks, along with little half-sandwich bags full of my own trail mix (raw almonds, walnuts, dried oat cereal, tart cherries, cocoa nibs, and the occasional wasabi pea). I portion out just one of those small bags. That's all I can have as my trail mix snack for the day.

For the first three days, I failed miserably, polishing off the entire bag before I left my kitchen. But over the next few weeks, I was able to make it last all day, knowing there would not be a second helping. (Psychological warfare!) That, along with fruit (apples and almond butter or a fresh fruit salad) and veggies (cut-up strips of any veggie with hummus or light cheese) got me through the day.

Moral of the story: Don't ever laugh at Joy or Erica.

#16
Befriend Fiber

SIMPLY PUT...Fiber should be a part of every meal or snack. If it isn't, find a way to sneak some in, either by substituting something on your plate with a fibrous food, adding a side dish that's rich in fiber, or sprinkling some in.

When I was younger, fiber was little more than *that thing that keeps you regular.*

I didn't understand the excitement my grandparents and their friends would always show when talking about it. Literally every one of their conversations would somehow steer itself toward fiber intake! I remember wondering as an innocent ten-year-old with a perfectly functioning digestive tract whether I'd grow up and sit around in circles with my friends and giggle and gossip about fiber the way Grandma and Grandpa did.

Well, fast forward a bunch of years and the answer is a resounding *sort of*...but for slightly different reasons. While fiber still boasts its old tag line of "it keeps you regular," there are so many more benefits I've come to know and love.

If fiber isn't sexy enough for you, think about it this way: Eating a meal or snack without fiber is like talking to someone with no personality who has nothing to say. Was it a conversation? Technically yes, but you end up walking away feeling empty. That's exactly what it's like to eat a meal without fiber. Here's why:

- Fiber fills you up faster.
- Fiber fills you up longer.
- Fiber curbs your hunger so you end up eating less.
- Fiber helps move things along inside your body, preventing you from absorbing as many calories from the foods you eat.
- Fiber stabilizes your blood sugar (so your energy and mood levels stay even and steady).

In a perfect world, everyone would be eating between twenty-five and thirty grams of fiber each day. (Also in a perfect world, my thighs would have been born in Thin City, all cold cereal would be calorie-free, and Michael J. Fox would have asked me to prom. He didn't…as if that needed to be said.) The truth is, when it comes to fiber, the majority of people out there are lucky to be getting half of what they should be getting every day.

But don't worry, that's probably not you.

By following the thirty Changes, you're probably already getting a decent amount of fiber through the foods you're now eating. But just in case, I'm going to have you effortlessly add a little fiber to every meal or snack. And we're not counting grams, I promise.

DON'T STOP THERE...

Look, if any meal or snack you're reaching for contains some sort of plant—whether it's something made from whole grains, fruit, or vegetables—then you're most likely getting some fiber. But if not (or you just want to maximize the benefits of this Change), there are plenty of ways to sneak in even more fiber without your palate noticing the difference.

There are the more obvious ones, like adding nuts or seeds to your meals, or eating brown or wild rice instead of white. But that doesn't mean there aren't plenty of other creative ways to sneak in more:

Need More Fiber?

Beans (cooked): If they seem like an obvious choice, you're right. You can look in the chart in this chapter (see page 110) to see how much fiber one cup of various beans brings to any salad, soup, sauce, or whatever you want to throw them on. But if you're looking for a bean that's less noticeable and less likely to roll off whatever you're putting them on, go with lentils—one tablespoon provides one gram of fiber.

Berries: Although the amount of fiber they bring varies depending on the type (see the chart in this chapter for an idea), any berry can raise your fiber intake significantly—so add away.

Carrot shavings: Grate a single carrot into a salad, on top of soup, or wherever you could use some orange to brighten things up, and you'll add nearly two grams of fiber into any meal without noticing a thing.

Chia seeds: Every tablespoon of these tiny seeds is packed with omega-3 fatty acids, but more important, a whopping five grams of fiber.

Cocoa powder: One teaspoon of unsweetened cocoa powder contains zero sugar but one gram of fiber. Try dusting it over your fruit (especially banana slices) or put some on top of a slice of whole-wheat toast with peanut butter.

Ground flaxseed: One tablespoon boasts almost two grams of fiber and it's versatile enough to be added to almost anything: yogurt, oats, soup, smoothies, cereal, a sandwich, you name it. (It even works great added into baked goods and used as a coating on chicken.)

Lima beans: Tossing on just a tablespoon of these green guys can punch up a meal almost a full gram of fiber.

Peanuts: A one-ounce serving (about 25-30 whole peanuts) can be sprinkled on practically anything, provides more than two grams of fiber, plus they're rich in heart-healthy monounsaturated fats.

Sesame seeds: A single tablespoon of this burger bun staple actually has one gram of fiber. Best of all, their nutty taste and crunch works on (or in) about anything you can think of.

Wheat germ or oat bran: Just one ounce of wheat germ contains about four grams of fiber (cooked oat bran comes in a little lower at one gram of fiber per ounce, but that's still not bad). Sprinkle either over the same types of foods you would throw ground flaxseed on, but don't let me stop you from being creative.

When Choosing, Go with Fiber

Choose almond or peanut butter over butter. One tablespoon of either adds one gram of fiber (regular butter has no fiber).

Choose uncooked oatmeal over breadcrumbs. Just a cup of dry oatmeal has eight grams of fiber (plus plenty of protein for your muscles). The next time a recipe calls for mixing in breadcrumbs (for hamburgers or meatballs, for example), switch it out. Or use dry oatmeal the next time you need to bread chicken or fish.

Choose rye over white. If you're eating bread during the day, whole grain is my top choice. But if you're not a fan, rye bread contains one and a half grams of fiber per slice—almost twice the amount you'll find in white bread.

Choose pie over cake. Even though I'd prefer you eat none of either, if you're left with no choice, pie (so long as it contains apple, cherry, or berries) is always the better option because you'll get more fiber.

Choose berries over whipped cream or syrup. If you are going to indulge, top your dessert or pancakes with sliced berries—the sweetness will satisfy as you add additional fiber to your treat.

Choose hearty greens over bread and tortillas. The next time you decide to make a sandwich wrap, use kale, chard, collard greens, Boston Bibb, or any other tough leaf you can roll up. You'll spare the carbs and calories while you boost your fiber.

Choose whole-wheat or vegetable-infused pasta over regular semolina. Both offer more vitamins, minerals, and fiber than the traditional kind—and have less effect on your blood sugar.

Choose mushrooms over meat. Opting for a thick portobello instead of a hamburger is an obvious move if you want to eat fewer calories. (You'll also get one gram of fiber for your efforts.) For something less extreme, try replacing a little (or a lot) of the meat in any meal that requires ground meat (like tacos or chili) with minced mushroom for an additional fiber boost.

Choose pureed fruit over jelly. Grab a high-fiber fruit like a banana, kiwi, mango, peach, pear, plum, papaya, or strawberry (or grab several different fruits), toss the fruit in a food processor, and whip it up. Spread it on your toast and you'll have something just as sweet as jelly with way less sugar and plenty of fiber.

Fiber You Can Mix In

Canned pumpkin: A single ounce delivers 1 gram of fiber, and its rather bland taste makes it easy to mix into everything without being detected, including protein shakes, your pancake mix, even a bowl of oatmeal.

Chopped onions: Five tablespoons of raw chopped onion can be thrown into an omelet, cup of soup, sandwich, or salad without even being noticed, but it brings with it a full gram of fiber.

Pears: Great for sweetening up a salad, shake, yogurt, or cereal, a single pear contains a whopping five grams of fiber.

Pureed vegetables: How much fiber depends on what vegetable you blend, but whipping up your veggies makes it easy to work them into a sauce or stew, giving it more bulk without affecting the taste.

Sauerkraut (low-sodium): One cup adds four grams of fiber, making it ideal for giving bulk to a meat dish, a sandwich, or any meal that would be complemented by its unique taste.

Sliced avocado: Rich in fiber, one half of this smooth, creamy fruit delivers about five grams. So stick it in a smoothie, chop it into a salad, put a slice on your burger or sandwich, or use it wherever you think the green guy would taste best.

A LIST OF SOME HIGH-FIBER FRIENDS		
Food	*Portion*	*Fiber (in grams)*
Acorn squash (cooked)	1 cup	9
Adzuki beans (cooked)	1 cup	17
All-Bran cereal	1/2 cup	10
Almonds	1 ounce	4
Apple	1 medium	4
Apricots (dried)	1 cup	9
Arugula	1 cup	0.4
Asian pear (raw)	1 fruit	4
Asparagus	3 spears	1
Avocado (raw)	1/2 fruit	9
Banana	1 medium	3
Black beans (cooked)	1 cup	15

A LIST OF SOME HIGH-FIBER FRIENDS (continued)		
Food	*Portion*	*Fiber (in grams)*
Blackberries (raw)	1 cup	8
Blueberries (raw)	1 cup	4
Boysenberries (frozen)	1 cup	7
Brazil nuts	1 ounce	2
Broccoli (cooked)	1 cup	5
Brown rice (cooked)	1 cup	4
Brussels sprouts (cooked)	1 cup	6
Bulgur (cooked)	1 cup	8
Cashews	1 ounce	1
Cauliflower (cooked)	1 cup	5
Collard greens (boiled)	1 cup	8
Corn (sweet white)	1 ear (large)	4

Food	Portion	Fiber (in grams)
Cranberry beans (cooked)	1 cup	16
Crookneck squash (cooked)	1 cup	3
Currants (red and white; raw)	1 cup	5
Edamame (frozen; prepared)	1 cup	8
Elderberries (raw)	1 cup	10
Endive (chopped)	1 cup	1.5
Fiber One bran cereal	1/2 cup	14
Figs (dried)	1/2 cup	7
Flaxseed	1 ounce	8
Garbanzo beans (cooked)	1 cup	12
Gooseberries (raw)	1 cup	6
Green beans	1 cup	3
Jicama (raw)	1 cup	6
Kale (cooked)	1 cup	3
Kidney beans (cooked)	1 cup	16
Kohlrabi (raw)	1 cup	5
Lentils (cooked)	1/2 cup	8
Lima beans (cooked)	1 cup	14
Mustard greens (cooked)	1 cup	5
Navy beans (cooked)	1 cup	19
Oat bran (raw)	1 ounce	12
Okra	1 cup	3
Orange	1 medium	4
Parsnip	1 cup	6
Peach	1 medium	2
Peanuts	1 ounce	2
Pear	1 medium	6
Peas, green, frozen	1 cup	14
Peas (split; cooked)	1 cup	16
Pepper (green or yellow)	1 medium	2
Pinto beans (cooked)	1 cup	15

Food	Portion	Fiber (in grams)
Pistachio nuts	1 ounce	3
Popcorn (air-popped)	3 cups	4
Prunes (dried)	1/2 cup	6
Pumpkin	1 cup	0.6
Radicchio	1 leaf	0.1
Raspberries	1 cup	8
Red cabbage (cooked)	1 cup	4
Red potato (flesh and skin)	1 medium	3
Rice bran (raw)	1 ounce	6
Russet potato (flesh and skin)	1 medium	4
Savoy cabbage (cooked)	1 cup	4
Sesame seeds	1/4 cup	4
Spaghetti (whole wheat; cooked)	1 cup	6
Spaghetti squash (cooked)	1 cup	2
Spinach (cooked)	1 cup	4
Starfruit (raw)	1 medium	2.5
Strawberries (raw)	1 cup	3
Sunflower seeds	1/4 cup	3
Sweet potato (flesh and skin)	1 medium	4
Swiss chard (cooked)	1 cup	4
Turnip greens (cooked)	1 cup	5
Walnuts	1 ounce	2
Watercress	10 sprigs	0.1
Wheat bran (raw)	1 ounce	12
White beans (small; cooked)	1 cup	19
Wild rice (cooked)	1 cup	3
Yams	1 cup	6
Yellow beans (cooked)	1 cup	18
Yellow squash (crookneck)	1 cup	2
Zucchini (cooked)	1 cup	3

Tips and Tricks

Even though this Change is pretty straightforward, there are still a few things to consider as you begin increasing the amount of fiber you're eating each day.

Don't shave off the skin. Eating fruits and vegetables with their edible peels intact boosts your fiber intake without trying, so even when you're slicing them up for the bowl you should now be keeping in your fridge, leave that skin on. The same rules apply for oranges, grapefruit, and other citrus fruits, but in a different way. Don't eat the peel (I had to tell you that?), but don't throw away the membranes that cling to the fruit when you peel them—they're also rich in fiber.

Let your belly be your guide. For some people, jumping into more fibrous foods can cause bloating, diarrhea, and excess gas. If that's you—and I think it will be fairly obvious to yourself, your immediate friends, and the poor guy who stood behind you waiting at the ATM if it is—then cut back the amount of fiber you sprinkle onto your meals and snacks by half to one-quarter until your body becomes used to it, then gradually build up the amount you eat.

If you're not sipping, you'd better start. As you increase your fiber intake, you need to be drinking plenty of water to help move fiber through your digestive system.

The "So You Know" Science

Fiber is a carbohydrate that your body can't break down, so it stays intact as it travels through your digestive system. It's found only in plants—in the leaves, stems, seeds, outer skin, and roots.

It comes in two types: soluble and insoluble. Soluble fiber—the type commonly found in barley, beans, oats, and some fruits such as strawberries and blueberries—dissolves in water and turns into a spongelike substance as it moves through your digestive tract. As it travels, it helps to stabilize your blood sugar by slowing down the absorption of carbohydrates into your bloodstream. It's also been shown to help slightly lower LDL (the bad cholesterol) and blood pressure.

The other type (insoluble fiber) is typically found in things like nuts, wheat and corn bran, whole wheat, brown rice, bulgur, and most vegetables, particularly the dark, leafy kind. Unlike soluble fiber, it doesn't dissolve in water, so it stays intact as it traps water and pushes things along, cleaning your digestive tract and keeping you regular as it goes.

#17
Switch to a 30-Minute Workout 3X a Week

SIMPLY PUT . . . Starting today, I want you to do some form of 30-minute full-body strength-training workout three times a week. You'll stop doing the workout from Change #10 (that 20-minute workout I showed you), but you'll continue to walk 10,000 steps each day.

(I'll pause for you to mumble out loud something about how it's crazy of me to expect you to work out an additional ten minutes *and* walk 10k steps. I can take it. But remember: If doing what you're trying to accomplish were easy, everyone would be doing it. And I can assure you, based on literally everything I know to be true, everyone is *not* doing this.)

Another actual phone conversation with my mom:

ME: Hey, Mom. Are you home?

MOM: Just walked in. Going to do my lunges before I get too tired.

ME: Oh, that's great! But didn't you just do lunges the other day?

MOM: Yup . . . every day for two straight weeks.

ME: *What!?!? Two straight weeks???* We talked about mixing things up!

MOM: I know, but I read an interview with J.Lopez and she did lunges to lose her baby weight.

ME: It's J.Lo.

If you're wondering why I'm changing things up a bit, then blame your body.

Whenever you do the same activity over and over again, your body starts to learn the most efficient way to do that activity so that it requires the least amount of effort. It's a survival mechanism to conserve energy, which was handy back when we all dressed in loincloths instead of layers and swung clubs for food instead of for birdies. But when you're trying to lose weight, that survival safeguard is more annoying than it is useful.

So change it up.

At the start of any new exercise routine, your muscles work as hard as possible because they don't quite know what they need to do yet. All that confusion causes them to burn a ton of calories trying to figure things out, but eventually, they do. It may not be all the way on autopilot, but it's pretty darn close.

Constantly changing things up will keep your muscles confused, and the longer they stay uncertain about what you're up to, the harder they work and the more calories you'll burn as a result. It doesn't take much. Even something as simple as mixing up exercises your muscles may already know in a different order can be enough of a tweak to shock them.

When I first started training a friend of mine (let's call her Marni, because that's her name), she had an entire routine set for herself at the gym: Her only form of cardio was a 45-minute spin class three days a week (because the timing worked with her kids' school schedule), and the only strength training she did was an abs class (because she didn't think she needed to focus on any other areas besides her midsection).

When I first started training another friend of mine (let's call him Lester Holt—again, because that's his name), he had a pretty steady gym routine. He went every day, but every day he did the same exact thing: push-ups, sit-ups, squats, and some form of cardio.

When I first started training a client of mine (let's call him Josh, even though his real name is Scott), he hated change in any form and basically just worked his chest from every angle. That's right—there are approximately 640 skeletal muscles in the human body. Josh/Scott was a fan of just the few that resided several inches below his chin.

All three put their time in, trained hard, and were committed to their fitness routines, yet all three weren't seeing enough results. Why? Because they were all doing the same routine day in and day out, so I sat down and redesigned their workouts to change things up.

With Marni, I had her suspend her gym membership, then started her off with a pyramid workout, which is a routine made up of ten bodyweight exercises that *anyone* (yes, even you) could do *anytime* (so it works with any schedule), *anywhere* (home, office, hotel, gym, park, mother-in-law's kitchen, boss's office—OK, don't do it in your boss's office), with *no* equipment whatsoever.

Each week, I gave her four different pyramids that took only ten minutes each to complete, swapping out various exercises to target different muscle groups, so that no two pyramids were ever the same. When we started, she could do only one without needing to stop. Today, Marni can do five in an hour, and that (along with additional cardio and strength training) helped her lose twenty pounds in eight months.

With Lester, I lowered the weight he was lifting, increased the amount of repetitions he was doing per exercise, and reduced his rest time in between exercises. I also added a few pyramids into his routine to increase his stamina, along with a series of plyometric moves (such as push-up claps and explosive squat jumps).

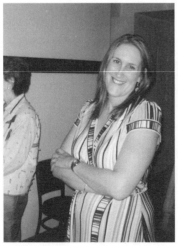
Marni, then

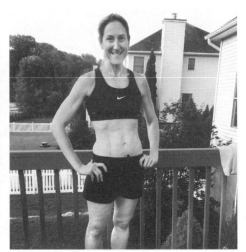
Marni, now

Within three months, he dropped weight, leaned out, and looked great. But more important, he now looks forward to new workouts every few months.

As for Josh/Scott, he still loves working on his chest, but I managed to get him to swap out most of his weight-lifting moves for some fun and functional plyometric chest exercises (such as throwing a medicine ball against a wall) and made him do a lower-body exercise immediately afterward without any rest. Once those tweaks were in place, he dropped weight and toned up pretty quickly. Is he still mildly obsessed with his beloved chest exercises? Of course! But he admits he loves how strong he's become since I switched up his routine.

Well…now it's your turn.

The Game Plan: Not only will you be changing things around, but as I mentioned at the start of this chapter, I'm going to be adding ten extra minutes to your strength-training workouts. This 30-minute full-body workout is composed of eight quick circuits of exercises that can be done anywhere—no weights or equipment required.

After each mini-circuit, you'll rest for sixty to ninety seconds, then move on to the next mini-circuit until you finish all eight mini-circuits. Again, you have a few options:

- You can do the workout once through as shown.
- You can do it once, then perform a 15-minute version afterward by repeating the routine but doing each exercise for half the number of reps.
- You can push through twice for a full 60-minute workout, but only if you find that the other two options aren't challenging enough.

Also, just like Change #10, there are no tips or tricks, but I still need you to remember a few things:

- Before every workout, do a quick five-minute warm-up. You can jog in place, walk in place while pumping your arms back and forth, lightly skip rope (or pretend to), or do any low-intensity activity that gets your blood flowing.
- Take one day off in between sessions to let your muscles rest and recover.
- Jennifer Lopez goes by J.Lo, or Jenny from the Block, but never J.Lopez.

THE WORKOUT

Mini-Circuit #1

(Do this circuit 3 times in a row)

- 20 fast mountain climbers
- 50 upper cuts

Mini-Circuit #2

(Do this circuit once)

- 40 wall push-offs
- 100 hip raises

Mini-Circuit #3

(Do this circuit once)

- 100 fast jogs in place
- 50 reverse claps
- 80 fast jogs in place
- 50 reverse claps
- 60 fast jogs in place
- 50 reverse claps
- 40 fast jogs in place
- 50 reverse claps
- 20 fast jogs in place
- 50 reverse claps

Mini-Circuit #4

(Do this circuit once)

- 40 wall push-offs
- 100 hip raises

Mini-Circuit #5

(Do this circuit 4 times in a row)

- 20 butt kickers
- A 20-second plank

Mini-Circuit #6

- 20 jumping jacks, immediately followed by 20 crab kicks
- 18 jumping jacks, immediately followed by 18 crab kicks
- 16 jumping jacks, immediately followed by 16 crab kicks
- 14 jumping jacks, immediately followed by 14 crab kicks
- 12 jumping jacks, immediately followed by 12 crab kicks
- 10 jumping jacks, immediately followed by 10 crab kicks
- 8 jumping jacks, immediately followed by 8 crab kicks
- 6 jumping jacks, immediately followed by 6 crab kicks
- 4 jumping jacks, immediately followed by 4 crab kicks
- 2 jumping jacks, immediately followed by 2 crab kicks

Mini-Circuit #7

(Do this circuit once)

- 40 wall push-offs
- 100 hip raises

Mini-Circuit #8

- 5 squats (on the last rep, hold yourself in the down position—thighs parallel to the floor—for ten seconds)
- 4 squats (again, pause and hold for ten seconds on the last rep)
- 3 squats (again, pause for ten seconds)
- 2 squats (and again, pause for ten seconds)
- 1 squat (that's right—pause and hold for ten seconds)

THE EXERCISES

Fast Mountain Climbers (see page 34)

Upper Cuts (see page 75)

Wall Push-offs (see page 39)

Hip Raises (see page 32)

Jogs in Place (see page 71)

Reverse Claps (see page 73)

Butt Kickers

THE MOTION: Jog in place, kicking your heels back toward your butt. (Kicking back each heel—left then right—counts as 1 rep.) If you can't get your heels to touch your glutes, just get them as close to each other as possible.

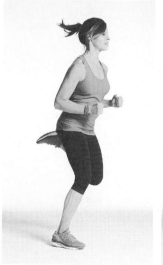
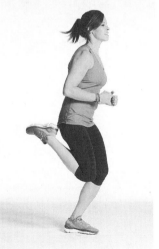

Plank

SETUP: Get in a push-up position—
legs extended behind you, feet
together with your weight on your
toes. Bend your arms and rest on your
forearms. I want your body to be in a
straight line from your head to your
heels.

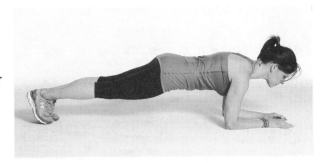

THE MOTION: There is none. Just hold the pose for the required number
of seconds.

Jumping Jacks (see page 72)

Crab Kicks (see page 31)

Squats (see page 36)

Don't Eat More Than Three Servings of Foods with More Than Five Ingredients

SIMPLY PUT . . . Look at the back ingredient label of every packaged food you eat and drink. Limit yourself to three servings daily of foods or beverages that have more than five ingredients in them.

An actual conversation with my mom

ME: Mom, your whole cupboard here is full of boxes of processed food. Look at these ingredients! There's gotta be twenty different words I can't pronounce here. Seriously, read this box.

MOM: Alkali, diglycerides, sodi...bicar...lychsomething...?

ME: OK, forget it.

MOM: But it's all low-fat...Does that count?

ME: No!! They're low-fat because of all the junk in them!

MOM: Well, how many ingredients do you want us to eat?

ME: Maybe three.

MOM: That's easy. Your father and I never have more than three at a time.

ME: Ingredients, Mom! Not servings!!

MOM: Oh.

Most people looking to eat healthier are so obsessed with the calorie, fat, and carb content in foods that they never bother to look at all their ingredients. And when they do, it's almost a joke to try and pronounce some of the things listed.

Sodium erythorbate?

Disodium guanylate?

Carrageenan?

Three words you'd think you'd find in a biochemistry class are actually a preservative, a flavor enhancer, and a fat replacer. (A fat replacer??? Did you even know there's actually such a thing?)

So ask yourself this: If you had a hard time *pronouncing* any of these three ingredients (or any ingredients in the foods you normally eat), why would you want to put them in your body? Think about that the next time you grab a box, bag, bowl, or bite of anything with a laundry list of ingredients. If you can't say them, why would you want to eat them?

And a lot of those ingredients aren't there to make the food healthier. Instead, they're typically preservatives, sweeteners, and other additives shoved in just to flavor, blend, thicken up, color, and/or mummify (ooh gross…mummify!) your food so it tastes great, looks pretty, and can sit unspoiled on a shelf decades (who knows, even centuries) from now.

Now, I could rattle off all of the ingredients in all of the foods in all of North America, but the Food and Drug Administration (FDA) already beat me to it with their database Everything Added to Food in the United States. (That's honestly the name and I'm honestly not kidding when I say, *"Really? That's the name?"*) It's a running list of more than three thousand food additives. If you have an extra year or two, check it out, it's a great way to spend the time (right up there with hailing a cab, changing a diaper, and watching paint dry). Fine, I'll spare you the details so you can focus on that number alone: 3,000!!!

Do you need to know them all to make the right choices with what you eat or drink? Absolutely not, since most of the concerns about food additives are aimed at the man-made ingredients added to foods. Examples are antibiotics, artificial dyes and sweeteners, nitrates, sulfites—you know, anything that was probably created in a laboratory by someone who had more diplomas than dates. (Don't get me wrong. I love diplomas.)

But the ingredients in healthy foods are almost always recognizable, never require a medical dictionary to understand, and most important, they're few and far between. Want a mashed potato? Make one from scratch and the only ingredient you'll see on the bag is *potato*. Make a box of instant mashed potatoes and enjoy the dozens of extra ingredients that come with it, such as calcium stearoyl lactylate and sodium bisulfite and FD&C yellow #5 & #6. (No snarky comment needed because I'm still trying to pronounce everything.)

From now on, you'll be picking more food with ingredients that make your mouth water—not wonder.

Your Plan

The only thing you need to do is look at the ingredients in whatever you're eating or drinking—that's all.

If there are more than five ingredients, then you can enjoy a serving (*one* serving) of the item. Limit yourself to three servings per day of any food or drink with more than five ingredients. Whether you spend that allowance on eating three servings of the same food or one serving each of three different foods, it doesn't matter. All I care about is that three is your limit for the day. By doing this, you will quickly see how easy it is to veer off track with this assignment. This will be challenging, but it'll be worth it as you start fueling your body with all-natural, healthy, *real* food.

DON'T STOP THERE...

If you could change your diet to the point where you're eating *only* single-ingredient foods, you would be my hero. Realistically, it's hard to avoid all the additives all the time. It's no secret at this point that my guilty pleasure is cold cereal. Put a box of Cinnamon Toast Crunch in front of me (make that any box of any cereal) and I'm putty in your hands. But I limit myself to sick days, pregnancy, and breakups. (Hopefully I'm done with two out of three of those.)

That doesn't mean you can't gradually tweak what I'm asking you to do to find a happy medium. If you want to challenge yourself even further, or feel such an impact from this Change after you implement it that you want to get even more from it, then you can try tapering down as you go in any of several ways:

- Reduce how many five-plus-ingredient foods you eat daily down to two, one, or none.
- Try eating only three servings of foods with four or more ingredients each day (then start tapering it down to three or two ingredients).
- Stick with eating only three servings of five-plus-ingredient foods on the weekends, but only two servings on weekdays.
- You get the idea…But again, if you stick with the original Change and that's all you ever do, you won't hear me complain.

Tips and Tricks

Eat any food in its most natural state and odds are, you'll never have to worry about any artificial flavors, colors, and preservatives disappointing you when you stare down the label. But having a little more information at hand can help you make the most of your five-or-less quest.

If it's in a box or bag, it's probably processed. Maybe not every time, but snack foods, white rice, regular pasta, cereal (sadly), instant oatmeal, and baked goods (including most pancake and waffle mixes) are usually packaged this way. The problem is that the carbs in these types of foods are typically made with refined grains—grains stripped of the good stuff (fiber) that can spike your blood sugar and cause you to store excess fat.

Go organic if it's an option. Organic fruits and vegetables may not always look as perfect, large, or tasty as nonorganic versions, but they have more vitamins and minerals—and none of the worries of chemical fertilizers and pesticides or wondering if what you're eating is a GMO, a genetically modified organism altered by science to take on particular traits (like needing less water to grow, or being herbicide resistant), which some fear could be behind certain health issues. Bonus points if you buy in-season foods that are locally grown.

Cook your own junk food. For those times when you really crave French fries, potato chips, cookies, cake, or any fried food, make it yourself. You'll not only be eating something that's void of additives, but you'll probably eat those types of foods less often because of all the effort involved.

The more convenient, the more you'll be counting. Ingredients, that is. Any food that calls itself *instant* or *ready-to-eat*—including frozen and pre-made meals—typically finds itself on the processed food list, bringing with it a bunch of additives. For the record, most fruits and veggies are also ready-to-eat—minus the additives.

If you don't recognize it—do your research. Whenever you read an ingredient you haven't seen before, make a habit of looking up exactly what it is. There are more than fifty different names for sugar, for instance, so what may seem harmless could be something you may want to avoid.

Think mini—not maxi. If you're going to keep a few five-plus foods around, buy the smallest serving possible, even if it's a single serve from a vending machine. That way, you're guaranteed to stick with only one serving. Buy the family-sized bag or box to save a penny and you'll only increase your risk of eating a bigger portion, or more portions than you should. It may be penny wise, but it's literally pound foolish.

If it claims it's "whole grain," look at the first ingredient. According to the Whole Grains Council (yes, this actually exists!), if the first ingredient listed contains the word *whole* ("whole-wheat flour" or "whole oats," for example), it's likely—but not guaranteed—that the product is predominantly made from whole grain. But know this loophole: If there are two grain ingredients, and only the second ingredient listed is a whole grain, the product may contain as little as 1 percent whole grain!

Go with foods you know won't keep for long. If it doesn't rot, there's a reason for it. Although honey is a rare exception to the rule, the longer something lasts in your kitchen, the more ingredients you'll probably find on its label. The more perishable foods you buy, the more likely you'll have no problem sticking with the three-servings-or–less rule.

Mix as many five-or-below foods as you like. Just because I don't want you to eat single foods with more than five ingredients doesn't mean you can't make foods with more than five—so long as the foods you're mixing together still qualify. For example, if you whip up a smoothie with four types of fruit, a little Greek yogurt, a tablespoon of peanut butter, and some chia seeds, what's in your blender will be well over five, but at least it will be additive-free.

If it's canned, rinse whenever possible. Nutritionists estimate that only about a quarter of your daily sodium intake comes from the salt you sprinkle. The rest is already inside the foods you're eating, which can lead to everything from bloating and hypertension to an increase in your appetite. To minimize the damage, try rinsing canned vegetables and beans before you cook or eat them—a trick that can reduce their sodium content by as much as 40 percent.

If it has trans fats, substitute it with something else. I don't care if it's a five-ingredient-or-below food, if you see the words *partially hydrogenated* or *hydrogenated*, it has trans fat in it. That means you're eating a molecularly altered unsaturated fat that boosts your levels of bad LDL cholesterol and lowers your levels of good HDL cholesterol. Worse yet: A label can still say "0 grams" of trans fat if the food contains less than 0.5 grams per serving.

To avoid them when cooking, try to switch to healthier monounsaturated oils (such as olive or canola oil). But if they're in any foods you love, see if you can find another version that's free of hydrogenated or partially hydrogenated oils.

#19
Eat Something Smart Before and After Every Workout

SIMPLY PUT ... Eat. Thirty to sixty minutes before you work out, have a small snack consisting of both protein and carbohydrates. Then, within thirty minutes after a workout, have another.

There's nothing more frustrating than meeting a client for a long morning workout only to hear them tell you they haven't eaten anything yet today.

ME: Nothing?
CLIENT: Nah.
ME: Why not?
CLIENT: Wasn't hungry.
ME: But you need something in your system to get you through the workout.
CLIENT: I'll be fine, trust me.
ME: OK, then let's start off with a quick hundred mountain climbers.
CLIENT: Um...OK. (*Pause*) Hold on...What's option B?

Your body is a machine. It won't run on empty. You shouldn't *want* it to run on empty, especially now that you're on your way to eventually exercising for a full hour. In order to work at maximum capacity, it needs fuel. The higher grade the fuel, the better results you'll see.

So what is high-grade fuel? It's a healthy mix of complex carbs and protein. In short, carbohydrates give you energy (so you can start a workout with 100 mountain climbers), and protein protects your muscles from being broken down to be used for energy and gives your body what it needs to rebuild muscle tissue that breaks down after exercise.

The key is not to overthink this. There are simple, easy, delicious snacks that work to satisfy your body's needs before and after a workout. Snacks that will help (not hurt) your waistline. Just something small and healthy that gives your body the right amount of what it needs—when it needs it.

DON'T STOP THERE...

You have undoubtedly heard every possible food theory out there...from every possible "professional" out there. Some will tell you your pre-workout snack should be relatively low in fat and fiber so it digests quickly, but that it should also be low in sugar so you don't get a surge of energy that peters out halfway through your workout.

Others might say that whatever you eat absolutely and positively has to be the perfect ratio of exactly 40 grams of carbohydrates to 20 grams of protein, eaten precisely one hour before you work out while standing on your head and counting to 300 in increments of 3½ (OK, maybe I exaggerated that last part).

Then there are those who will swear you need to switch to easily digestible carbohydrates (such as white bread or fruit juice) so your body can use those carbs immediately. And also that when carbohydrates are synthesized from carbon dioxide and water using light as an energy source, it's photosynthesis.

What?? Must. Turn. Back. Way too complicated...brain hurts!

Look, if it requires too much mental work, you won't stick to it. The truth is, you don't need all that noise. For right now, I don't want you counting calories, calculating percentages, or obsessing over grams of protein and carbs in meals. If you were a bodybuilder, or someone training for an athletic event, then you and I would be having a different conversation altogether—but that's not what this is all about. I just want you to eat something relatively healthy before and after your workouts. And that's it.

Need Some Suggestions?

Personally, I have my own favorite go-to pre- or post-workout snacks. Here are my top three in no particular order:

- Hummus with cucumber and tomato slices on whole-wheat pita
- Oatmeal or yogurt with slivered almonds and low-fat chicken sausage
- Baked sweet potato topped with 1 percent cottage cheese

However, there are so many combinations you can try, depending on your tastes, time, and whatever's easiest for you to grab. Here are just a handful of snack combos you can use to refuel and rebuild your body—both before and after the hard work:

Instant Eats

- One piece of fresh fruit and either a small glass of milk or a whole hard-boiled egg
- One serving of plain low-fat or nonfat Greek yogurt topped with either a handful of granola, berries, whole-grain cereal, or almonds
- One handful of dried fruit and nuts
- One glass of nonfat or low-fat chocolate milk
- One or two sticks of low-fat string cheese and a piece of fruit
- A small bowl of any whole-grain cereal and one cup of low-fat or skim milk
- A slice of whole-wheat toast covered lightly with almond butter
- One-third cup of chickpeas with a squirt of lemon juice (or eat the same amount roasted if you like them crunchy)
- A half cup of cottage cheese topped with a handful of chopped up fruit
- One serving of cheese and a handful of carrots
- One medium apple and two tablespoons of all-natural peanut butter
- One or two handfuls of either dried or steamed edamame and a piece of fruit

Mix-'Em-Up Meals

- Blend 1 scoop of vanilla protein powder, 1 cup of orange juice, and ice.
- Blend ¼ cup of unsweetened almond milk, ¼ scoop of protein powder, ½ a banana, ½ tablespoon of almond butter, and ice.
- Blend 1 scoop of chocolate protein powder and 1 cup of iced coffee.
- Blend 1 scoop of vanilla protein powder, ½ cup of cherries (fresh and pitted), ½ cup of low-fat or skim milk, 1 tablespoon of honey, and ice.

A Little Work, but Worth It

- A small serving of oatmeal and either ½ glass of milk or a hard-boiled egg
- Two or three slices of low-sodium deli meat on a slice of whole-wheat bread with honey mustard
- Mix up 3 ounces of chicken breast (chopped), a few avocado slices, and ½ cup of cooked whole-wheat pasta
- One serving of light tuna salad (made with hummus instead of mayo) and a handful of whole-grain crackers
- One frozen waffle (any kind) with 1–2 teaspoons of almond butter
- A deck of cards–sized piece of roasted turkey and an equal-sized portion of sweet potatoes or brown rice
- One brown rice cake with ¼ avocado and a hard-boiled egg on top
- One half of a whole-wheat pita filled with ¼ cup of hummus
- A small bowl of fruit, plus scrambled eggs or an omelet (using 2 or 3 eggs maximum) mixed with a handful of chopped bell peppers, onion, spinach, or any other veggie you like

Tips and Tricks

It's hard to give any more advice than asking you to eat. However, there are still a couple of things for you to keep in mind (or try) that may help:

If you exercise at noon, split up your lunch. Working out over your lunch break? Try splitting up what you would normally eat into halves. Eat one half, exercise, then finish your lunch once you're done.

Don't wait longer than thirty minutes to eat post-workout. Your body's ability to process glycogen—the stored energy your body uses as fuel when you exercise—is at its highest right after exercise. Eating within that window will leave you with more energy for the next day.

Watch your intake of "performance water." Just because it says "water" on the packaging doesn't mean it's good for you. Most are loaded with sugar, which will only keep you from losing weight by adding unnecessary calories. That goes for sports drinks too.

Don't assume you can eat more than necessary. Many people tend to overestimate the amount of calories they've burned while exercising, leaving some feeling that they have the freedom to eat anything and everything afterward. Remember, it's a post-workout *snack* (not a meal), so keep it light, between 200 and 300 calories.

The "So You Know" Science

If you think that eating before and after a workout feels like taking one step forward and ten steps back, here's why it's crucial.

Right after you exercise, your body's main goal is to replace its inventory of glycogen and rebuild your muscles. It turns to whatever food it can find in your system first, but if there isn't anything to convert, it may begin to eyeball your muscles. By not eating carbohydrates both before and after exercising, your body can fall into a catabolic state where it begins breaking down all your hard-earned muscle to convert into glycogen.

Another reason that carb/protein snack is important is because every time you strength train, you're actually creating microscopic tears within your muscles. Once you're through exercising, your body immediately starts looking for amino acids to rebuild your muscles. If your belly's empty, it has to wait until you finally feed it something it can use, which can delay how fast your muscles recover and hold back your results.

#20

Make at Least Three Everyday Activities More Challenging

(Or as I like to call it...burning calories without actually working out)

SIMPLY PUT ... Pick a minimum of three activities, tasks, or errands you do every day and find a way to make them a little more challenging so you'll burn more calories.

A few years ago, a friend of mine kept complaining (and complaining and complaining) that she had no time to go to the gym because of work (and the long commute and the hours and being tied to her desk and seven hundred other things). So about a half mile before my wit's end, realizing that an explanation alone wouldn't be enough to convince her that all that noise was just an excuse, I decided to *show* her instead.

So I got a heart rate monitor and made her wear it for an entire day—from sunup to sundown—to show how many calories she could burn without ever having to step foot in a gym. If you know me, you're aware that when I commit to something, I fully commit: I packed a bag and spent the night at her place, so that we'd be ready to go the next day.

At 6:00:00, the alarm went off.

At 6:00:04 (give or take a centisecond), we went to work.

We strapped on the heart rate monitor and immediately knocked out 25 squats while she was brushing her teeth and another 25 waiting for the coffee to brew. We did a couple of wall push-offs in the elevator while leaving her building, balanced on each foot at the subway stop, then got off a stop early from her job and walked. Even on the job, I had her doing biceps desk presses in her office (explained later in this chapter), triceps dips using her desk chair (also explained later in this chapter), upper cuts while on a conference call, a few lunges on her way to lunch, and a few more wall push-offs on the back of her door afterward.

By 1:00 p.m. she had already burned 300 calories. By the time she went to bed that night, she was up to 700 calories and had put in a full-body workout without stepping foot in the gym, taking a minute away from her job, or having to put on any workout clothes.

That was the last time I heard her complain about having no time to exercise.

Look, are there days when I don't get to the gym? Of course there are. Are there days when I don't work out? Never. I just have to get a little creative on those non-gym days, which, as you just read, isn't that hard to do.

The problem is that it's in our nature to want to make the easiest choice possible. It's in our nature to do things quicker and more efficiently.

Texting your kids from the kitchen that dinner's ready instead of walking upstairs to tell them is the easy thing to do.

Waiting for the next big rainstorm to wash the dirt off your car instead of getting outside with a bucket and sponge and doing it yourself is the easy thing to do.

Stuffing all of your laundry into one basket so you only have to make one trip upstairs instead of three is…yes, you got it…the easy thing to do.

Don't settle for easy. Let everyone else do that.

These are all wasted opportunities to do something good for yourself. They are free gifts that burn additional calories but cost nothing and require no preparation. So think about everything you do, everywhere you go over the course of the day, and choose three things to challenge yourself with.

DON'T STOP THERE...

When it comes to this Change, open up your mind to all possibilities, because there are millions of ways to challenge yourself more out there, even if you never leave your home.

Whenever I'm emptying the dishwasher, I squat down, grab a single glass, plate, sippy cup, or whatever else just ran through the rinse cycle, and stand up before putting it where it belongs. Would it be easier to bend at the waist and grab as many things as humanly possible to save time? Obviously. But instead, I'll squat down and grab just one because I know I'm working my entire lower body and burning a few extra calories.

That's one of a hundred examples of ways to create calorie-burning scenarios. All you need to do is avoid looking for the easiest way from point A to point B. Instead, it's time to find the more scenic route and make whatever it is you're doing more interesting, active, challenging, or fun.

Once you get the hang of it, you'll start to find that you won't settle for just making three activities more challenging. If you exceed that number, I'm happy. So long as whatever you're doing never cuts into your time to finish your 10,000 steps each day (or your strength-training sessions), then the more the merrier.

Tips and Tricks

There are countless ways you can do this, but here are a few obvious—and some off-the-wall—ideas that can get you thinking about how to do it.

Trade in the mop for some elbow grease. Any house chore you hate doing is probably one that requires a little hard work—and blasts a few extra calories. If you're 140 pounds, ten minutes' worth of light cleaning burns off about 27 calories. Just ten minutes! But take your cleaning seriously and you'll burn even more: 37 calories at a moderate pace and 48 calories if you clean at a vigorous pace.

Other suggestions:

- When wiping counters, surfaces, and appliances, switch arms to give both an equal workout. (FYI: Removing soap scum really tones your arms.)

- When unloading the dishwasher or hanging up clothes, squat down for each item instead of bending over to pick up several items at once.
- Before putting groceries away, grab a bag, lift it in front of you to shoulder height, and then bring it back down to your waist. Do 15 of these with each bag before unloading it.

Make the most of your office space. There are times for all of us when work has us so crazy we want to run around in circles out of sheer frustration. The good news—you'll burn off some calories. The bad news—you'll look silly doing it, especially if you work in a tiny office.

Other suggestions:

- *Paperclip squats*: Drop a bunch of paperclips on the floor. Squat down and pick up each one individually.
- *Triceps dips*: Place your butt on the edge of your desk, palms on either side of you. Bend your elbows as you slowly come off the desk and dip down a few inches, then push back up. Aim for three sets of 10 to 15.
- *Biceps work*: Sit at your desk and place your palms under the desk facing up. For thirty seconds, push up on the desk as hard as you can to engage your biceps. Do three sets of 30.

Wall push-offs (see page 39.) Aim for 35 to 50.

Be noble instead of needy. If you're ever in a situation where there are limited seats and you have the choice to sit or stand (on the bus or subway, at a party or concert), give up your seat and stand instead—you'll burn an additional 30 to 50 calories per hour for being courteous.

Other suggestions:

- If possible, invest in a standing desk.
- Count the number of steps from your car or subway to your office and increase it by ten every day by finding a longer route.
- When on the phone, get up and pace.

Use a basket instead of a shopping cart. Carry one or two baskets (one for each hand) when shopping. As you walk around, just squat down to place both baskets on the floor, stand back up to grab what you need, squat back down to put it into a basket, then lift both off the floor and keep shopping. It may take you an hour to shop, but think about your glutes!

Make every meeting an opportunity. Instead of just meeting a friend for coffee, or going out for dinner on a date, get creative and meet to do something active, whether it's going for a run together, hitting a climbing wall, playing tennis, or anything that gets your heart rate up and lets you socialize at the same time.

Be the "playdate" house. Unless your kids only have friends who are extremely tidy (they don't), opening your house up for a playdate is a guarantee that things will get messy and displaced. After the fun's over, you can offer to help clean up with them.

Have a stand-to-squat rule. Whenever you're stuck standing for short periods of time—like brushing your teeth, waiting for the microwave to ding, or blow-drying your hair, for example—squat down an inch or two, hold that position for a few seconds, then stand back up. The move is so subtle that even if you're in public, no one will notice you're doing it, but you'll be conditioning your butt, thighs, and calves with every dip.

Rethink your rooms, then reorganize them. Moving furniture around may be a hassle, but it's a hassle because it takes effort—64 calories' worth every ten minutes!

Sweat through the commercials. Whenever you're watching TV, make the most of the commercial breaks by picking one of the following five exercises without stopping until your show comes back on.

1. Squats (see page 36)
2. Hip Raises (see page 32)
3. Upper cuts (see page 75)
4. Kneeling Push-ups (see page 40)
5. High Knees **The Motion:** Standing with your feet hip-width apart and arms bent at 90 degrees, quickly raise your left knee as high as you can, lower it back down, then quickly raise your right knee as high as you can and lower it. That's 1 rep. Keep alternating without stopping.

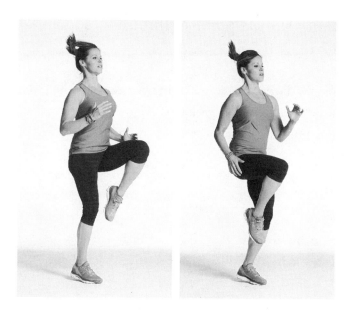

Shrink the size of your tools. Instead of grabbing the largest rake, broom, or shovel you can find when cleaning up leaves, sweeping the floor, or shoveling snow (or doing any chore where using a larger tool can help you save time), pick a tool that's as small as possible. You'll still get the job done, but it will force you to spend more time burning calories to do it.

The "So You Know" Science

Running, cycling, and aerobics are popular activities when trying to lose weight, but cardiovascular exercise is actually any activity that raises your body's need for oxygen. Once that happens, your heart and lungs start working harder than usual to deliver that oxygen, and your body ends up burning calories as a result.

Despite what may be trendy, your body doesn't care what activity or task increases its oxygen need. It could be pushing your kids on a swing, raking leaves, or chasing after someone's serve on the tennis court. The only three things that matter to your heart are frequency (how often you challenge it), intensity (how hard you push yourself), and time (how long you keep it challenged for).

Any activity that elevates your pulse to between 50 and 70 percent of your maximum heart rate (MHR)—and keeps it there—will do the trick. (To find your MHR, just subtract your age from 220.) But if you don't have a heart rate monitor, use this tactic:

- If you can talk during the activity but singing would be too difficult (or you can get a few words out, then have to stop talking to take a breath afterward), your pulse is probably somewhere in the range of 50 to 70 percent of your MHR.
- If it's easy to speak long sentences as you go, you're most likely not doing anything at a pace that's keeping your pulse in that 50 to 70 percent zone—so step it up.
- If you're unable to talk, then be careful, because you're pushing yourself too hard and more than likely have a pulse that's above 70 percent of your MHR.

#21

Make an "I Will Do" List and Stick to It

SIMPLY PUT...Write out a to-do list of everything you need to do tomorrow. Take two of those items off that list and move them to a new list—the things you WILL do tomorrow. No matter what happens—those two things *must* get done.

There are two kinds of people in the world—those who say I SHOULD and those who say I WILL.

I used to be an I SHOULD girl. My days were always filled with things like: I should go work out; I should order the salad; I should finish up this paper before I go out tonight; I should try yoga, call my mom, eat more broccoli, ask him out, ask *her* out. I can go on, but I'll spare you my boring to-do lists from days/months/years past. (Although "ask *her* out" isn't a boring story at all...but I digress.)

Then about fifteen years ago, I met my friend Bill. He was an I WILL guy—charming, successful, charismatic, and driven. My parents loved him (as dating material) and never wasted an opportunity to tell me so. Truth be told, there wasn't much *not* to love.

Bill was fun to watch. He was like a machine when it came to getting things done every day. He would take a 6:00 a.m. spin class, read three papers, walk his dog, do errands on his way to work, call, text, and e-mail everyone back, order groceries, arrange furniture deliveries, have his front hall painted, book a vacation…and then he would stop for lunch.

As a perennial I SHOULD girl, this was obviously incredibly annoying to me. While I was having a hard time just sitting down to *write* my to-do list, Bill was knocking off his and anyone else's in a ten-mile radius. So one day (read: one of my particularly unproductive days), I asked him his secret.

"There's no real secret," he explained. "Just try not to prioritize certain things over others on your to-do list. Don't always stick 'work' on top. Don't always drop 'gym' to the bottom. And if that's where they belong, then switch up the list every few days."

I was sold.

That same I SHOULD girl who used to prioritize her to-do list based on what she felt was most important (work on top, paying bills somewhere in the middle, and on the bottom: work out, eat more vegetables, and cancel my extra AOL e-mail account— Hey, I said it was years ago!) eventually became an I WILL girl. I quickly realized that the people who always seemed to find time to get everything done *never* had more time in their day than I did—they just knew how to prioritize better.

The takeaway? *Everyone gets the same twenty-four hours a day, seven days a week.* It's what you do with that time that matters most.

I WILL vs. I SHOULD

Instead of creating a traditional to-do list, I want you to imagine two separate lists: One is I WILL DO and one is I SHOULD DO.

The I WILL DOS are the things we never falter on because we either love to do them or we know the consequences are too great if we don't do them:

- I WILL get up in the morning, brush my teeth, get dressed, go to work.
- I WILL watch my favorite TV show.
- I WILL be at that two o'clock meeting.
- I WILL get my kids up and ready for school.
- I WILL pay my bills.
- I WILL take the garbage out every week.

And then there are the I SHOULD DOS. These are the tasks we know we need to do, but when push comes to shove, they're the ones that get the big heave-ho:

- I SHOULD organize my workspace better.
- I SHOULD go back to yoga and take my bike out of storage.
- I SHOULD fix that squeaky door that drives me crazy every time I open it.
- I SHOULD get to those 156 e-mails in my inbox.

Prioritizing your life in the right order is a crucial step within the thirty Changes. Being able to keep priorities in your life from stacking up reduces stress because it will mean there's one less thing you need to worry about.

But more important, it will remind you that you're on top of—and in control of—your day, which will leave you feeling more accomplished, motivated, and energized. It's that positive feeling that can boost your pride and help you make smarter decisions as the day goes on, which will make sticking to the thirty Changes much easier.

Your Task

So, each day I want you to make a list of everything you need to do for the next day. Then take two of those tasks (preferably two you feel are the hardest to stick to) and move them to your I WILL DO list. I need you to make whatever those two tasks are just as important as brushing your teeth, taking the kids to school, and earning a paycheck—so they get crossed off your list for good.

The fewer things left on your plate, the less stress you'll feel in your life, and the easier it will be to stick with the thirty Changes.

DON'T STOP THERE...

Even though I'm hoping that you've performed all of the twenty Changes you've learned so far to the letter—and that you'll do the same with the Changes about to come—I'm not naïve. I know there have been several you've probably stumbled with along the way.

Was it the twenty sips of water first thing in the morning? Or did the cold weather last week make it easier to pass on the 10k steps for a few days? Look, only *you* know which Changes have been an easier journey than others, so I want you to make me—no, make yourself—a deal.

I'd like you to take whichever few Changes seem to be the hardest to stick with and move them to your I WILL DO list. Some healthy lifelong habits take a little more work than others, and the more often you can cross them off your list, the more they will become part of who you are.

Tips and Tricks

Everyone has their own methods for keeping themselves on track. But there are a few proven approaches that can make decision making and task management a little easier. If you're having a hard time turning an I SHOULD into an I WILL, then give a few of these a try.

Never write vague goals—write specific actions. Jotting down goals that are too broad and unclear (like "clean the upstairs") can feel too imposing. Even if you managed to clean half of it, not being able to check it off your I WILL DO list at day's end can leave you feeling defeated. Instead, write down only specific tasks (such as "vacuum the upstairs bedroom" or "put away all the towels in the upstairs bathroom," for example) that are immediately actionable.

Create your own "maximum capacities." Clutter is killer, and having too many things—whether its e-mails or tasks you've taken on—can leave you feeling buried. Instead, use the two-for-one rule: Before you allow yourself to take on something new, make yourself finish two things that have been sitting around waiting for your attention.

Don't be afraid to say no. Just as no one likes a yes-man, being a no-thank-you person may seem like you won't earn any points with friends. But always being generous of your time when people are constantly interrupting your day to gossip—or asking you to help them with *their* to-dos—can make it impossible to address your own.

Don't be a multitasker—be a single-tasker. Despite how proud spinning twenty plates at the same time may make you feel, most people are far more productive focusing on one task instead of dividing their focus between several.

It's OK to jump from one task to another, but always give whatever task you're working on your absolute attention.

Write out a "to-don't" list. We all have those little habits or distractions or vices we pour time into while getting little back in return. If you know yours, scribble them down. (Mine tend to include spending too much time with my four social friends, Twitter, Instagram, Facebook, and Pinterest.) Then copy that list several times so you have one in view by your desk, in your car, in your kitchen, taped to your iPad—anyplace where seeing a list of your time eaters will guilt you into not wasting away your day.

#22
Eat Something Every Two to Three Hours

SIMPLY PUT . . . Eat. I want you to have breakfast and then follow it up with small meals every two to three hours, so that you never feel hungry at any point of the day.

Why do diets fail? They fail because we get hungry, because we don't like to be deprived, and because we always want what we're told we can't have. Diets fail because self-control doesn't always apply when pizza, fresh baked bread, wine, and dark chocolate–covered pretzels are sitting around. So what can you do?

Avoid getting hungry. We'll get back to this in a moment.

Any new parent will tell you: Once your kids are on a set sleep schedule, your life becomes a bazillion times easier. (Actually, is there a number higher than a bazillion? Because that would be it.)

The day you can put your child down and they *go* down, and they *stay* down, and they wake up at roughly the same time every morning, is a day that every parent dreams of. Why? Because the uncertainty is finally over—and a schedule is born.

When things happen *on* schedule—whether it's at your job, on vacation, in your house, at the airport or bus terminal—everybody gets what they want and the world's a beautiful place. (Did I go too far? Trust me—if you're a parent, you understand.) When things are *off* schedule, people become frustrated and make impulsive decisions. You are left feeling tired and unfulfilled, looking for shortcuts.

Well, your body is just another big stubborn baby that needs to be on a schedule too. When you eat meals or snacks infrequently, your body questions if (or when) it's going to be fed again, and it can throw a massive tantrum that puts most two-year-olds to shame.

Anytime you wait too long between meals—or miss a meal altogether—your body can interpret that innocent slipup as starvation, which can cause it to break down lean muscle tissue for energy and store a greater amount of whatever you eat during your next meal as fat. It's not your body's fault. It doesn't always know, so it holds on to things it's not always supposed to hold on to. Worse yet, that big baby can throw a fit in the form of cravings for even larger amounts of food later in the day.

But when you can get yourself on some semblance of a food schedule (by simply eating every few hours at predetermined times), your body begins to learn when it's going to get food next, making it less likely to send you hunger signals or make you crave more food than you need to eat. But even better than that, it's less likely to hold on to excess calories.

Getting your body on a food schedule is fairly easy. It's as simple as waking up and eating breakfast. After that, have something to eat—a healthy, smaller meal or snack—every two to three hours from that point forward.

So a typical schedule might be:

7:30 a.m.: Breakfast
10:00 a.m.: Snack
12:30 p.m.: Lunch
3:00 p.m.: Snack
5:30 p.m.: Dinner
8:00 p.m.: Snack

Once you figure out what works best for you, do you *have* to eat only at those times? No—none of this is foolproof or absolute. And sticking to a perfect food schedule isn't something I would expect to happen every single day. But breaking up your daily calories into smaller meals will pacify your inner baby. Plus, digestion burns calories, so by eating more frequently, you'll keep your metabolism elevated longer throughout the day. (And just to be clear, this isn't a green light to eat for twenty-four straight hours. That's gross.)

DON'T STOP THERE...

Are there ways to get even more from this Change? Absolutely, but it does take a little more effort than just eating more often. If you're serious about eking out everything this Change has to offer, there are several ways to do it:

Make breakfast the most important meal of the day. There are not many things that I will force you to do, but this is one of them. Even if you're not a breakfast eater, I really need you to have a little something first thing in the morning, and you can start very slowly.

Look, I'm not telling you to sit down and have the lumberjack stack. I just want you to remember that when you wake up, your body hasn't eaten for the longest period of time of your entire day. It's burned through most (or all) of its stored glycogen, so it's looking for calories.

If you don't send any calories down by eating breakfast, your body is heading for your muscles instead, breaking down what you've worked hard at building up. Even if you never wake up starving, if you wait hours to eat after getting up, once you finally do eat something, your body will hang on to those calories for dear life. So start your day with a little something to satiate you.

Try to balance every meal and snack. Ideally, each one should contain one serving of protein, one serving of carbs, and one serving of healthy fats. To be more specific:

1. *A serving of a lean protein* (from low-fat meat, fish, or dairy products—if you're vegan, tofu is fine too)
2. *A serving of a complex carbohydrate* (from fruits, vegetables, or certain grains, such as brown rice, oats, or quinoa)

3. *Some type of healthy fat* (which may already be present in your protein—cold-water fish have plenty of essential fatty acids, for example—or may be added through other sources, such as nuts, seeds, or certain types of oils, like olive, canola, or sunflower oil)

Why all three? Protein, carbs, and fats are digested at different speeds. Carbs are digested the fastest, protein takes a little longer, and fats take the longest. When you eat all three in the same meal or snack, it gives you a steady stream of energy that keeps you from feeling hungry between meals and snacks and prevents your blood sugar from spiking (so your body never releases as much insulin, which can cause you to store fat).

If you slip up, don't starve yourself. Will there be times when you don't manage your meals right and end up eating more than you should? Hopefully not, but if it happens, don't punish yourself by skipping your next meal. Just go back to eating the same-sized meals and your body won't enter panic mode.

Finally…Don't overthink it!!! My little culinary secret is that I don't cook. It's not that I don't love to eat, or that I don't appreciate good, healthy food—I just never really found my way around the kitchen. Ask anyone I've ever dated.

Even when I try, I fail. I failed eighth-grade home economics because I was assigned to make spaghetti and I didn't know I was supposed to boil the pasta! I just took dry spaghetti, broke it into pieces, and put it right in the sauce. True story. Pathetic, but true.

As a result, to this day, I don't use/own/read recipes and I avoid math at all costs. So giving me five recipes and asking me to eat 35 percent of this and 25 percent of that is all lost on me.

This is all my way of saying I don't ever, ever overthink my meals.

I don't want you to have to think about them all the time either. In Change #15, I showed you how to eyeball your portions with your hand when preparing your meals, so you always know what a normal serving size looks like.

If you look down and see a serving of protein and a serving of complex carbohydrates each time you eat, I'm happy. And if you're not eating fatty fish rich in omega-3 fatty acids (such as salmon or tuna), then add a thumb's worth of healthy fats by sprinkling on some nuts or drizzling in some healthy oil.

If that sounds too difficult, let me show you how easy it is to pull together something tasty that mixes all three in one shot:

Some Breakfast Ideas

- A serving of plain (unsweetened) yogurt with raspberries and ½ a whole-wheat bagel
- A whole-grain English muffin with 2 to 3 ounces of smoked salmon and a slice of tomato
- A serving of oatmeal (mixed with raspberries and a teaspoon of flaxseed oil) and a glass of low- to no-fat milk
- A spinach omelet (3 egg whites and 1 whole egg, mixed with a handful of baby spinach) with a piece of fruit
- An egg-white omelet (3 to 4 egg whites with ½ cup of diced vegetables thrown in) and ½ a grapefruit
- A cup of plain nonfat yogurt (mixed with ground flaxseeds and a few strawberries) and a piece of 12-grain bread
- A whole-grain waffle, a glass of skim milk, and a handful of blueberries
- Two slices of whole-wheat bread with a tablespoon of peanut butter and a glass of skim milk
- A serving of unsweetened whole-grain cereal (with a cup of skim milk and a few walnuts mixed in) and some grapes

Some Lunch Ideas

- A whole-wheat pita filled with homemade tuna salad (made with 1 can of spring-water tuna, ¼ cup of low-fat mayo—or oil and vinegar—and some shredded red bell pepper)
- Three ounces of chicken breast, cut up and mixed with 1 cup of whole-wheat pasta and drizzled with olive oil, with a side of mixed greens
- Three ounces of fresh turkey breast or chicken breast on rye bread (with lettuce, tomato, and onion), and ½ cup of mixed berries mixed with sunflower seeds

- A 3-ounce lean hamburger and a slice of Swiss cheese tucked inside a whole-wheat wrap with dark-leaf lettuce, a slice of avocado, a slice of tomato, and a little mustard

Some Dinner Ideas

- Three ounces of shrimp, 1 cup of chopped mushrooms, peppers, and onions (grilled on skewers), ½ cup of quinoa, and 1 cup of mixed greens (with a drizzle of olive oil)
- Three ounces of grilled salmon, 1 cup of cooked long-grain rice, and 1 cup of steamed asparagus
- Three ounces of grilled chicken, ½ cup of couscous (with shredded almonds mixed in), and 1 cup of steamed snow peas
- Three ounces of filet mignon on a bed of arugula with chopped tomatoes and sliced avocado
- Three ounces of top round steak, 1 medium-sized sweet potato, and 1 cup of broccoli drizzled in olive oil
- Three ounces of bottom round, 1 yam, and 1 cup of broccoli mixed with almond slivers

Some Snack Ideas

Some of the pre- and post-workout suggestions I gave you in Change #19 are also great mini-meals and snacks that you can turn to even on days when you don't exercise. And here are a few more you can try out for size:

- One cup of low-fat cottage cheese, mixed with 1 cup of raspberries and some sunflower seeds
- A hard-boiled egg with ¼ sliced avocado on whole-wheat toast
- Two slices of low-fat cheese and 2 slices of either fresh-sliced roast beef or turkey breast (rolled up inside each other), with 1 ounce of almonds
- A sliced pear covered in one serving of almond butter, and a glass of skim milk
- Fat-free Greek yogurt with almond slivers (I always carry a little ziplock bag of almond slivers with me to sprinkle on yogurt and oatmeal when I'm

on the road. They are a good source of protein, magnesium, potassium, vitamin E, and fiber.)

- An apple and reduced-fat string cheese (portable, easy to eat, and healthy!)
- A bag of grapes with 2 hard-boiled eggs or rolled-up turkey slices

Today show Tested

As glamorous as network news is often made out to be, it really isn't. (Sorry network news, but you're not.)

It's busy and unpredictable and exhausting. Every day, you're assigned a different story in a different city at a different time. How can you possibly keep an eating schedule when you have no idea where you'll be or for how long? And there's nothing worse than fishing around at the bottom of your bag in sheer hunger for anything edible, only to have to settle for a half-eaten protein bar from months ago, which is now hard as a rock. (And the answer is yes, shamefully I would have eaten it.)

When Lester Holt, Erica Hill, Dylan Dreyer, and I all kept food diaries together (and e-mailed them to one another every night), we got a chance to see not only *what* we were all eating, but *when*. And the *when* turned out to be the more telling story.

If Lester was off on a *Dateline* shoot, he could go eight hours without eating. Sometimes Dylan would have a little breakfast treat in the early morning and then not eat again all day. Erica and I were a little more consistent, but not by much.

So one thing we all tried to improve on after a month of sharing our diaries and analyzing our eating patterns was *when* we ate. We tried to focus on breaking up those two or three big meals into smaller, healthier, more frequent meals.

Erica and I emptied the NBC commissary of slivered almonds and Greek yogurt, the perfect "in-between meal" snack. For Lester, it meant grabbing chocolate milk (a great source of protein and carbs) after his workouts when he was running late. (There's nothing cuter than a well-dressed man with a high-powered job on television drinking a little box of low-fat chocolate milk.) Dylan made breakfast at home and brought it with her if she was sent out on a weather story.

Bottom line: We were all prepared and rarely starving. After a month, we actually found that our dinners were all smaller portioned when we ate more consistently throughout the day. (And FYI, if anyone runs into Lester at a bar and wants to buy him a drink: chocolate milk.)

#23
Rethink What You Drink

SIMPLY PUT . . . Before you drink anything that isn't water, check how many calories it contains, then ask yourself two questions:

- "Do I want to *drink* these liquid calories or would I rather save them and eat something filling instead?"
- "What am I really craving right now?"

I promised you I wouldn't have you counting calories, but that doesn't mean I want you to ignore that they exist.

A lot of people feel that if they aren't chewing their calories, then they're not ingesting calories. Well, I hate to break it to you, but calories are calories, whether they come from the foods we eat or the beverages we drink.

When you start adding up what you quenched your thirst with over the course of the day—that glass of orange juice with breakfast, a whole milk latte for the car ride to work, a soda with lunch, a glass of wine at night—these are all calories that you could've avoided. Or at least saved and used to eat more nutrient-rich foods.

Even worse, most liquid calories tend to be empty and nutrition-less, particularly alcohol, coffee, and soda. Even beverages you may assume are healthy for you—like energy drinks or fruit juice, for example—are not as rich in nutrients as their whole-food counterparts and are oftentimes packed with sugar. All that sugar triggers the release of insulin, which causes your body to store more excess calories as fat.

But the biggest reason to watch what you're drinking is because you can drink faster than you can eat. You can't chew what you're drinking twenty times until your stomach catches up, so it's easy to throw back a lot of calories without even realizing it. And when people drink beverages with a lot of liquid calories, they also tend to eat a lot more calories with them.

What makes this Change so powerful is that by cutting back on your "liquid calories," your body will never notice the difference. Since liquid calories don't satiate hunger (only thirst), by trimming them back rather than cutting back on your calories by eating less food, you don't experience the same feelings of deprivation. If you're already hydrated, craving liquid calories is usually nothing more than a need for taste—but it's usually not anything you can't satisfy in other, less caloric ways.

Your Plan

I'm not expecting you to go cold turkey on what you drink, but instead to keep liquid calories from making your journey more difficult. Try doing the following things before you take that first sip:

1. Look at the calorie amount of what you're about to drink, then ask yourself if you could benefit more by spending those calories eating something. Would I prefer to see you trade in the 200-calorie caffè latte you usually throw back to wake up in the morning for a four-egg-white omelet, a piece of fruit, and a big cup of black coffee? Let's all say yes at the same time.
2. Ask yourself, "What am I really craving?" Whenever we reach for something to drink, there's a reason for it. Are you just thirsty, or are you craving something sweet? Is it the carbonation that you're looking for, or is it just having something warm to sip? You may be surprised that what you crave is something that could just as easily be found in other, non-caloric options like a cup of hot tea, some seltzer water (with a hint of lime), or plain old water.
3. If all else fails, pick the smallest size possible. Everyone loves a bargain, but whenever you bump a drink up from small to supersize to get more

for your buck, your body is paying for it later. Going with the smallest size possible is usually enough to satisfy your taste buds without having to disappoint your waistline.

Need an idea of what you might be adding to your day? This general list of the most commonly reached-for drinks will give you a ballpark tally on how many calories you're tacking onto your daily total without realizing it:

Beverage	Serving Size (ounces)	Calories (on average)
Alcohol (80-proof gin, rum, vodka, whiskey), minus any mixers	1.5	100
Apple juice (unsweetened)	12	170
Beer (regular)	12	150
Beer (light)	12	100
Carrot juice	12	150
Chocolate milk (whole)	12	300 to 320
Chocolate milk (2%)	12	285
Chocolate milk (1%)	12	230 to 240
Coconut water	12	60 to 70
Cranberry-apple juice	12	225
Cranberry juice cocktail	12	200
Cranberry juice (unsweetened)	12	165
Caffè latte (with skim milk)	12 (tall)	100
Caffè latte (with whole milk)	12 (tall)	205
Cappuccino (with whole milk)	12 (tall)	110
Coffee (black)	12	0 to 5
Coffee (with two Tbsp. of 1% milk or skim milk)	12	25
Coffee (with two Tbsp. of half-and-half)	12	60
Cosmopolitan	2.75	150
Grape juice (unsweetened)	12	225
Grapefruit juice (either pink or white)	12	130 to 145
Green tea (either bagged or loose)	12	0
Milk (whole)	12	220
Milk (2%)	12	180

Beverage	Serving Size (ounces)	Calories (on average)
Milk (1%)	12	155
Milk (skim)	12	120
Mineral water	12	0
Orange juice	12	160 to 180
Piña colada	9	490
Pineapple juice	12	200
Pomegranate juice	12	200
Seltzer or sparkling water	12	0
Soda (diet)	12	0 to 10
Soda (regular)	12	120 to 190 (depending on the brand)
Tea (unsweetened)	12	0 to 5
Tomato juice	12	60 to 70
V8 vegetable juice	12	75
Wine (red)	5	125
Wine (white)	5	120

Tips and Tricks

For those times when nothing will do but a hot cup of this or a cool glass of that, considering a few clever switches before you swig could make those liquid calories feel a little less shameful.

Reverse your java habits. Coffee by itself has zero calories—it's the stuff you're mixing into your cup that's the culprit. So before you pour yourself coffee, take a teaspoon or tablespoon (depending on what you're pouring into your coffee) and add what you typically put into your cup or mug first. (Milk, cream, sugar, donuts...whatever!) Being able to see what you're actually adding can help you make smarter choices—or lessen the blow.

Here's an idea of what you're adding to your coffee with each and every spoonful:

- Agave nectar: 20 calories per teaspoon
- Granulated sugar: 16 calories per teaspoon
- Half-and-half: 20 calories per tablespoon
- Heavy whipping cream: 52 calories per tablespoon
- Honey: 21 calories per teaspoon

- Liquid concentrate creamers: 25 to 35 calories per tablespoon
- Milk (skim): 5 calories per tablespoon
- Milk (whole): 10 calories per tablespoon
- Whipped cream: 8 calories per tablespoon

Substitute a second cup with something different. Instead of pouring another coffee after you've had your first, switch to something else warm but even better for you, such as steeped ginger root or green tea, instead. You'll start to realize that a second cup of coffee isn't needed as much as you think.

Pulp it up over plain. If you can't live without having a glass of fruit juice, then at least burn a few calories grabbing some fresh fruit and using a hand juicer to squeeze out a glass on your own. All the effort could make you appreciate what you've poured a little more (so you won't be as likely to just chug it back), plus it adds more pulp, which leaves you feeling more satiated.

Add a splash of seltzer or water to any juice. Instead of pouring a full glass of juice, leave some room at the top and pour in some seltzer or cold water—preferably filtered so adding it doesn't change the taste. Diluting your juice a bit won't ruin your drink, but it will spare you a few calories for the effort. As you get used to the taste, try cutting back a little at a time until you're fine with drinking a mix of half juice and half seltzer or filtered water.

If you're dying for a smoothie, roll up your sleeves. Making your own smoothie (instead of having one made for you at your favorite juice bar franchise) will give you control over what's being whipped up. It may take more time and effort, but you'll most likely add fewer calories, which will save you time sweating them off later on.

To keep your fruit smoothie under your caloric budget, these low-cal veggie options add plenty of bulk to your blender, have zero to little flavor (so you'll still taste whatever fruits you're mixing together), and are fortified with vitamins, minerals, and fiber.

- Bok choy
- Cabbage
- Canned pumpkin

- Celery
- Cucumber
- Jicama
- Spinach
- Summer squash
- Tomato
- Zucchini

Choose a lighter option, but pretend it's regular. Going with a lower-calorie version of a drink is always a better choice—but it can also cause you to drink more because you feel less guilty. The problem: Many low-sugar drinks are sweetened artificially, using ingredients such as aspartame, saccharin, sucralose, and stevia. What you may save in calories you might make back by eating more, since some artificial sweeteners may also increase your appetite.[1]

Have one or two water chasers for every alcoholic beverage. Will you be peeing every few minutes? Probably. But here's the thing: Alcohol has 7 calories per gram. (That's more than carbohydrates, which have only 4 calories per gram.) It also triggers the release of insulin to help break down the excess sugars found in most alcoholic beverages, which can lead to any extra calories from alcohol being metabolized and stored as unwanted body fat. Added bonus: Staying hydrated also lessens your chances of experiencing a hangover!

Consider a siesta over a Red Bull. Most energy drinks are not only loaded with calories, they typically contain ingredients I dare you to recognize—let alone pronounce. If a boost of energy is what you need, opt for a plain coffee or tea instead, or give your body what it really needs—a quick nap.

Today show Tested

As hard as this is to believe, I never had coffee before joining the *Today* show back in 2007. It wasn't a caffeine thing—I just didn't like the taste of it. And no, it's not lost on me that as a non–java drinker working on an early morning show, I'm a walking, talking oxymoron.

So you could imagine my frustration when, shortly after getting in and settled at NBC, I realized that a ton of business (meetings, deals, interviews, chats, gossip, run-ins, and discussions) took place over coffee runs, specifically at the Starbucks at 30 Rock, where our offices are. Without a coffee drink to purchase (and I don't do tea), I was odd woman out.

Nobody wants to have a grown-up conversation in grown-up clothes at a grown-up job with a girl who orders a hot chocolate, but "hold the whip."

One day, on a business trip to Detroit, my producer Lindsay (who was tired of hearing me "hold the whipped cream") decided it was time for me to dive into the wide world of java. So we stopped at an airport coffee shop by our gate, ordered about ten different drinks (I'm not sure everyone in line that day appreciated our little experiment) and tasted each drink until I found something I could muddle my way through well enough to sit at the grown-up table.

It honestly wasn't until that very moment that I actually took the time to look at the calories on some of the drinks. As a non–coffee drinker, I had no idea some of them packed such a fat punch! A hundred, 200—even 400 calories for a coffee drink?? I could understand if it was sold in an edible croissant cup—but 400 calories!! Yet the lines at every coffee house around town remain endless.

Despite a lot of these places displaying calorie counts on beverage menus now, the mocha, frappé, whipped, creamy, frothy, syrupy, sugary, triple-shot, three-pump, vanilla, quad venti full-fat latte cappuccino drinks (or at the least some version of those) are still the rage.

In case you're wondering, I settled on an Americano with a little steamed nonfat milk. It's low calorie, packed with caffeine, and sounds so cool to order.

And while I was late to the table—the coffee table, that is—you should see the way my legs spin wildly, like a cartoon character darting for the door, when anyone asks to discuss something over coffee.

#24
Do a 45-Minute Workout 3X a Week

SIMPLY PUT . . . Starting today, I want you to do some form of 45-minute full-body strength-training workout three times a week. You'll stop doing the workout from Change #17 (the 30-minute workout I showed you), but you'll continue to walk 10,000 steps each day.

It's all about progression. Just when you get used to something, you have to shock the body and kick it up a notch. The change will make your muscles work harder. The harder work will burn more calories. The more calories you burn, the happier you'll be. The happier you are, the more you'll stick to the program. And the longer you stick to the program, the happier I'll be. So it's win-win!!

All kidding aside, what I'm building you up to is a full 60-minute workout. That's how long *my* workouts are. That's how long my clients' workouts are. You can do everything and anything in sixty minutes: cardio, strength training, balance drills, flexibility movements, core work, speed work, homework (OK...not homework).

Can you still do a lot in less time? Of course! There are days I have only ten or twenty minutes free, and on those days I pack the workouts with as much as I can. But you never need more than sixty minutes and that's where we're heading. But first, a stop at forty-five minutes.

First of all, I know you can do this. It won't be easy, but none of the truly rewarding things in life are ever easy. It's called a *workout* after all. Not a chillout. Not a hangout. Not a relaxout. Not a grab-a-beer out. And not a grab-a-book-and-kick-your-feet-up out (unless it's *this* book). It's a workout, so put the **work** in and you'll get the results **out**.

But if adding another fifteen minutes to your three-times-a-week workout sounds like a lot, just know that the hardest work is already behind you. The exercises you've been doing since we began haven't just been moves that build lean muscle and burn fat. They've been teaching your muscles to work together in a way that improves your functional strength, coordination, and endurance. That's been the harder adjustment to make along the way. Now you're ready for the fine-tuning.

Will this routine be a little more challenging for you? Obviously. But it's supposed to be. When the workout is no longer a challenge, it's time to move on and switch things up.

But aren't you also in a little bit better shape than you were before we started this journey together? Don't you have a little more energy as a result of eating better and reducing your stress? Haven't you started to lose a little weight? Don't you like what you're starting to see? I know the answer is yes to those questions, which is why this is the Change that's going to help take you from satisfied to electrified.

The Game Plan: This new workout takes only about twenty-two to twenty-three minutes to complete, but you'll be doing it twice, so that your total workout time will reach forty-five minutes. The entire full-body workout is composed of only five quick circuits of exercises, all of which you're already familiar with from previous chapters.

Why no new moves? You won't need them. The exercises you've already been doing are some of the most effective bodyweight exercises around. So instead of giving you new moves, I'm giving you new ways to *do* the moves. Changing the length, intensity, or rest time between sets each makes an impact, and for this Change, you'll be doing all three.

There are five mini-circuits made up of various exercises. You'll go through the exercises without resting (or with minimal rest). After each round, you'll rest for only one minute, then move on to the next mini-circuit until you've completed all five.

Once you're finished, you have a few options:

- You can do the workout again for a full 45-minute workout.
- You can repeat the workout 2 more times for a full hour-plus workout.
- You can just do the workout once and stop right there, but only if you've been using the book as a 30-Day program—and this is Day 24—and your body isn't quite ready yet.

Depending on your level of fitness when you started this program, you may—or may not—be ready to move from a 30-minute routine up to a 45-minute workout, and that's fine. But if that's the case, and you feel you can only do this routine once, I still need you to build up to being able to do the workout twice through. Keep going back to it and see if you can do a little more each time.

Just like Change #10 and Change #17, there are a few rules you must follow to make sure your muscles are prepared for every workout:

- Before each workout, do a quick five-minute warm-up.
- Take one day off between sessions to let your muscles rest and recover.

THE WORKOUT

Mini–Circuit #1

(Do this circuit 5 times in a row)

- 20 jumping jacks
- 20 front kicks (left leg, right leg = 1 rep)
- 100 upper cuts (left fist, right fist = 1 rep)

Mini–Circuit #2

(Do this circuit 4 times in a row)

- 20 high knees (left knee, right knee = 1 rep)
- 50 shoulder circles (forward)
- 50 shoulder circles (backward)
- 50 quad drops

Mini–Circuit #3

(Do this circuit 3 times in a row)

- 50 butt kickers
- 15 slow mountain climbers
- 50 apple pickers

Mini–Circuit #4

(Do this circuit 2 times in a row)

- 30 pikes
- 25 squats

Mini–Circuit #5

(Do this circuit 1 time)

- 50 jumping jacks, one 10-second plank
- 50 upper cuts (left fist, right fist = 1 rep), one 10-second plank
- 50 high knees (left knee, right knee = 1 rep), one 10-second plank
- 20 slow mountain climbers, one 10-second plank
- 20 squats, one 10-second plank
- 20 pikes, one 10-second plank

THE EXERCISES

Jumping Jacks (see page 72)

Front Kicks (see page 78)

Upper Cuts (see page 75)

High Knees (see page 136)

Shoulder Circles (Forward) (see page 71)

Shoulder Circles (Backward) (see page 71)

Quad Drops (see page 76)

Butt Kickers (see page 119)

Slow Mountain Climbers (see page 34)

Apple Pickers (see page 30)

Pikes (see page 33)

Squats (see page 36)

Plank (see page 120)

Tips and Tricks

Once you devote yourself to a 45-minute workout three times a week, every little bit helps. Here are a few things to think about—and try—that could help you get even more from the extra time you're now putting in.

Feel the burn—but keep your cool. You'll be able to comfortably exercise longer and harder if you stay cool, as opposed to letting yourself get too warm, which can lower your performance by placing stress on your body's thermo-regulatory system. Try to cool down the temperature wherever you are as you burn calories.

Grab your phone and record your routine. The more familiar you become with the exercises in this book, the easier it can sometimes be for your body to reposition itself to make the exercise easier to perform. If your form isn't perfect, you could be cheating yourself out of results. Recording yourself from certain angles, particularly from the side and from behind, will allow you to play the routine back and look for exercises you may not be doing properly in the heat of the moment.

Try a new room—or take it outside. Just because you'll be using the same routine several times a week doesn't mean you have to perform it in the same place twice. To keep it fresh, mix it up and do your workout in a different place each time whenever possible. If you're stuck in the same place, even facing another direction can help each workout feel slightly different.

Don't expect to improve every single session. The more you exercise, the fitter you'll feel and the stronger you'll become. But that doesn't mean that with every workout, you can always expect to see and feel an improvement compared to the last time. Just keep in mind that your progress may ebb and flow, but the longer you stick with it, the fitter you'll become.

If you exercise before bedtime, know this: For some people, working out right before going to bed can help them have a much deeper, restorative sleep. But revving up the metabolism through a long workout can leave some people feeling more alert, which could keep them from getting enough shut-eye. If that's you, try to schedule your workouts earlier in the day.

Today show Tested

After weeks of talking to my good friend Lester Holt about his workouts (tons of push-ups, ridiculous amounts of abs, and lots of biking), I invited him to do one of mine. When he asked me about it, I left it pretty vague: a 60-minute, boot camp–style workout that combined cardio work, strength training, plyometrics, and balance drills. (OK…maybe it wasn't *that* vague.) After a few seconds of silence, he asked, "Do any of those words include abs? I like doing abs." I assured him we'd be doing tons of core work, which, yes, included abs.

We met that Friday morning at the gym as planned. NBC has an incredible gym in the building. It's so convenient, and always fun to see colleagues out of their work mode and into their work*out* mode. (I won't name names, but that Stephanie Gosk is one fast runner!!) And as always, Lester was right on time and ready to work. (He's so ridiculously punctual and so pleasantly perfect all the time—yes, exactly as he is on TV.)

I knew this would be a more intense routine than he was used to. I figured there would be some growing pains, but we still dove right in with a few of my tougher circuits. And while it seemed like a bus ran over him, and then backed up and ran over him again, he pushed through the entire 60-minute workout. (Love that guy!)

Why was this workout similar to his, yet so hard? The exercises weren't that *different* from the ones he was already doing—but I did change three things about them. We did them longer, I added a second (and sometimes a third) muscle group to each move, and I took out the rest time between exercises, all to improve his stamina, stability, and strength.

That one Friday workout turned into a standing appointment every week. And every single week that followed, we built in even more changes to make each workout harder. Eventually Erica Hill, Dylan Dreyer, and Natalie Morales all joined in, each coming in with their own different and unique athletic backgrounds (some runners, some spinners, some just Lester). And they all pushed themselves for sixty jam-packed minutes and walked away realizing that if you love how you work out, you don't have to change it completely to make it more challenging.

Sometimes, just a few tweaks are enough to see and feel a real difference.

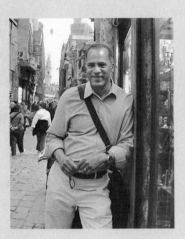 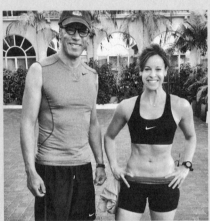

#25
Drop or Reduce Added Sugar

SIMPLY PUT... Women should limit themselves to no more than six teaspoons (that's about 24 grams, or 100 calories worth) of added sugar a day. And men, your limit is nine teaspoons (or about 36 grams—150 calories worth) daily.

Three weeks. That's it.

Three weeks is about how long it takes to get rid of a craving. If you can commit to three weeks, you can drop your craving for sugar. If you drop your craving for sugar, you can drop a dress size or two. If you can drop a dress size or two, you can drop by your ex's house to subtly show off the new you. If you can drop by your ex's house...Just do me a favor and drop added sugar.

Three weeks doesn't seem like a long time, does it? As with kicking any craving, *starting* is the hardest part, followed by *sticking with it* and then *not cheating*. And while I'll admit that reducing added sugar is difficult, it's also doable and could very well prove to be the most important and impactful of all the Changes you make.

Why is sugar so hard to break up with? Well, for one thing, candy tastes good. (Thank you, Captain Obvious!) So does chocolate. And don't forget cake, cookies, pie, pastries, frosting, batter off the beaters, whipped cream straight from the can, mini and mighty white chocolate morsels, gummies, anything that starts with *ice* and ends with *cream* or *flan*. But I don't have to tell you that all those delicacies come at a high price.

Forget about sugar leaving you overweight and toothless! Eating too much of it also makes you more susceptible to a slew of chronic illnesses ranging from diabetes to heart disease. So trimming back on the stuff is something you should have seen coming to some degree—but there's only one problem.

It's impossible to cut sugar out of your diet completely, since it's found in pretty much everything you eat, whether naturally or added in as flavor. That's why I'm asking you instead to reduce your intake.

Naturally occurring sugars—the type you find in dairy products, fruits, vegetables, and whole grains—are fine. Do some fruits and veggies have a greater impact on your blood-sugar levels than others? Yes, but the vitamins, minerals, and fiber that come with them far outweigh the amount of sugar in them. Besides, you would have to eat an obscene amount of food to have dangerous levels of sugar from any of the above. Nobody ever got a sugar high from eating too many apples.

Added sugar on the other hand—the kind they put into foods—is another story. You don't need it, it's addictive, and it's one of the worst things you can put into your body. It gives you worthless empty calories that contain few to no nutrients.

To make matters worse, since most high-sugar foods also have little to no nutritional value (think about it—do you ever remember anyone talking about how rich in fiber tiramisu is?), you're probably missing out on eating more nutrient-rich foods.

The more sugar you eat, the more addictive it becomes and the harder it is to silence your sweet tooth. But if you eat less, the opposite happens. You'll discover that you become more accustomed to eating less—and find that smaller amount to be just as satisfying. Try it. The less sugar you use, the less you'll *want* to use.

Your Plan

Because of the twenty-four Changes put in place up until this point, you've already made some lifestyle modifications that should be curbing your cravings for sugar. Eating lean protein in the morning, never skipping a meal, getting enough rest, and even exercise, all help minimize your desire for the sweet stuff.

But now that you're ready to reduce your sugar intake for good, there are a few things you need to consider:

Know it by its many tricky titles. Just a few common names for added sugar to watch for (and believe me, you'll be grateful for this list down the road):

- Agave nectar or syrup
- Barley malt
- Beet sugar
- Blackstrap molasses (great name for a band!)
- Brown sugar
- Cane juice (or sugar or crystals)
- Caramel
- Carob syrup
- Coconut sugar
- Corn sweetener
- Corn syrup
- Dextran
- Fruit juice concentrate
- High-fructose corn syrup
- Honey
- Invert sugar
- Malt sugar
- Maltodextrin
- Maple syrup
- Molasses
- Raw sugar
- Rice syrup (or brown rice syrup)
- Sorghum
- Sugar molecules ending in *-ose* (dextrose, fructose, galactose, glucose, lactose, maltose, and sucrose)

- Syrup
- Turbinado

And that's not even all of them! Why so many names? Because by going by more than fifty different names, sugar can hide itself wherever it wants. Annoying, right? All those names make it easier for food companies to prevent the word *sugar* from ever popping up at the top of the ingredient list.

Here's how they fool you: Some foods will use *smaller* amounts of *different* types of sugar to add sweetness. Each may seem insignificant because they're all placed low on a food label's list of ingredients due to their individual size. But when combined, their total volume can end up making sugar the main ingredient of whatever food or beverage you're having.

Stop drinking your sweets—and you could cut your sugars in half. According to a recent report by the 2015 Dietary Guidelines Advisory Committee, sweetened beverages are behind 47 percent of the US population's added sugars intake. In fact, sip down one twelve-ounce soft drink and you'll have thrown back an average of ten teaspoons of sugar, which exceeds the daily limit of added sugar for both men and women. So stay away from sugary drinks of all kinds.

Instead of substituting—scale back. Sugar substitutes (a.k.a. artificial sweeteners) can be tempting as a great replacement for table sugar, since they don't raise your blood sugar or trigger the release of insulin. But even though some are made from natural sources (such as stevia leaf extract) instead of synthetically (such as aspartame and saccharin), they may still cause adverse side effects.

Depending on which sweetener you reach for, it may have been shown to make medications less effective, decrease healthy gut bacteria, or slow down your metabolic rate. Moreover, it could contribute to insulin resistance, a risk factor for diabetes. The concentrated sweetness can also make you less interested in naturally sweet healthy foods and cause you to gain weight by intensifying your cravings for sugar and/or making you feel as if you can eat more and not gain weight because you're eating something with low to no sugar content.

Tips and Tricks

Whether you're looking for smarter ways to feed your sweet needs or wish you had more advice on how to keep sugar at bay, these tips can make lowering your sugar fix a much smoother process.

Know where secretive sugar likes to hide. You already know the obvious places, but don't ignore the not-so-obvious places. Just a few sneaky spots you will find a lot more sugar than you might expect include:

- Baked beans
- Barbecue sauce
- Coleslaw
- Dried fruit
- Flavored yogurt
- Granola
- Instant oatmeal
- Jellies and jams
- Ketchup
- Protein bars
- Salad dressing
- Spaghetti sauce
- Sweet pickle relish
- Tomato soup

Mix something sweet with something unsweetened. The same trick I suggested a few chapters back, of mixing fruit juice with water, also works with sugary foods. If you have to indulge, get creative blending things together, like making a half-and-half mix of no-sugar BBQ sauce and regular sauce, plain yogurt with sweetened yogurt, or chopped tomatoes and plain tomatoes with bottled pasta sauce. As you get used to the taste, start changing the ratio by adding less of the sugary stuff.

Find what's behind your craving. For many, reaching for sugary things is less about taste and more about seeking comfort or a reward. Before you nibble on sweets, ask yourself why you're doing it. If you're feeling sad, anxious, or proud, you could be feeding that emotion instead of eating for taste.

Pick your meat wisely. Even though beef, eggs, fish, and pork are naturally sugar free, anything that's marinated, cured, flavored, or processed (lunch meats, for example) may contain surprising amounts of sugar.

Don't always believe the package. Seeing "Without Added Sugars" or "No Added Sugar" on a food's package only means no sugar was added during processing. It still may contain significant amounts of sugar or be sweetened with fruit juice concentrate (which contains natural sugar).

If you can't go cold turkey—then dial back to start. Again, sugar is an addiction. But if cutting all the way back to twenty-four or thirty-six grams is a major struggle, I'll let you slide and start with forty-eight grams (whether you're male or female). Since the average American consumes about twenty teaspoons (or eighty grams) of sugar daily, you'll still be starting at just over half that amount. Eat one teaspoon (four grams) less each week after that until you reach twenty-four or thirty-six grams.

Spend your daily sugar on something healthy. Don't just blow your daily allowance of sugar on a soda, or waste it on the hidden sugars in dressings, sauces, or something you wouldn't find on any dessert list. Saving that allowance for a small special treat may make avoiding sugar all day long less painful.

Cut back on sugar when cooking. If a recipe calls for sugar, cut it back by one-third to a half. (You probably won't even notice the difference, but just in case, you could try cutting less to start.) Or, when possible, substitute something else for the sugar, such as an equal amount of unsweetened applesauce or pureed fruits such as figs, dates, apricots, or extra-ripe bananas. (Just be sure to add a little water to any puree before you add it to your recipe.)

Be experimental with a few extracts. It doesn't matter what flavor you prefer—almond, lemon, maple, mint, orange, or vanilla—using an extract rather than sugar (whether in a recipe or just to flavor up something when what you really need is a little sweetness) can do the trick, minus the excess sugar—or calories!

The "So You Know" Science

I'm not the only one who's sugar strict. The World Health Organization lowered their sugar-intake recommendations from 10 percent of your daily calorie intake to

5 percent (roughly six teaspoons a day).[1] The American Heart Association doesn't ask you to do the math, but suggests the same amounts that I'm asking you to limit it to: six teaspoons for women and nine teaspoons for men.[2]

Eat more than your fair share—and the average American consumes more than two to three times that amount—and you're exposing your body to a lot more than obesity. You get the lion's share of all the health risks that come with carrying too many pounds, including high blood pressure, diabetes, cancer, and osteoarthritis. According to research, ingesting too much sugar also increases your risk for kidney stones, promotes inflammation, lowers your good cholesterol (HDL), and raises your bad (LDL) cholesterol levels, increasing your risk of heart disease.

#26
Perfect Your Posture

SIMPLY PUT . . . Check your posture all day long. Be mindful of proper positioning: Your head should be up and looking forward, your spine should be straight, your shoulders back, and your ears in line with your hips.

Nowhere is posture more front and center than on TV, when you're on full display. And having worked morning, noon, and night shifts, I found the early morning time slot to be the toughest on your posture.

The *Today* show had been the ultimate posture check for me. I was always on early in the morning (when my body was tired and wanting to hunch over). I'd usually wear a tight, sleeveless dress (unforgiving to slumping shoulders), and the camera angle was often a full-body shot (to fully accentuate good/bad posture).

You really have to work to maintain that straight, lean look, especially when they attach an audiobattery pack (not small, by the way) to your bra (not a joke, by the way), resulting in that never-sexy hunchback look. So while the cameras were rolling, we would all overemphasize our posture—shoulders way back, neck super high, spine long and lean.

The minute we were off the air, we would all collapse like Shrinky Dinks!

So what does *good posture* mean—and why should you care?

Tilting your hips too far back, rounding your shoulders, or bending your neck may not seem like a big deal. But any (or all) of these things ruin your posture. The more centered your spine and joints are, the easier it is for your body to work the way it's supposed to—as efficiently and effectively as possible.

Spending hours hunched over a desk or walking around with your neck angled down as you type away on your handheld device places stress on certain muscles. It can also compress your lungs, preventing them from drawing in enough oxygen. The end result can be constant muscle fatigue and soreness, loss of stamina, and a higher risk of injuring yourself.

But when your posture is flawless, it lets your body eliminate unnecessary motions as you move, so it can perform the same tasks with the least amount of effort and fatigue. For your body, that means less pain and stress on your muscles and ligaments. Plus, it doesn't hurt that standing straighter makes you look taller and thinner…so there's that.

That's why before I start a training session with a client, I always do a posture check. I have them stand against a wall with their feet about six inches away. I make sure their head, shoulders, and butt all touch the wall. Then I try to squeeze my hand in between their lower back and the wall, and again between their neck and the wall. If there's only about an inch of space between the two, it's posture perfect. If there's more, we've got work to do.

So why are we a society in need of some spine straightening? Answering that question is never easy because there are so many ways over the course of a lifetime that our bodies fall out of good posture: taking a bad fall, poor sleeping habits, being overweight, knee problems, hip problems, weak muscles, sitting at your desk all day, text neck (looking down while typing), stargazing (staring up), ant watching and/or looking for lost change (staring down). It all adds up, leaving most of us looking—and feeling—off balance.

By incorporating the thirty Changes, you're already making lifestyle choices that will improve your posture naturally. Changes such as silently strengthening your core, using a workout that trains your muscles evenly to prevent muscular imbalances, and reducing your stress (which can prevent excess muscle tension) all help your posture and keep everything in alignment. But that doesn't mean you're free and clear.

Having perfect posture isn't impossible, but it does take a little bit of imagination. *Whenever you're standing or walking, imagine there's a balloon above you with a string that's tied to the top of your head, pulling your body upward.*

Just thinking about that image should be enough of a nudge to help get you back into alignment. But if you want to see how well it works, have someone take a picture of you from the side. Ideally, your ears, shoulders, and hips should all be in alignment with one another. If they're not, keep trying. With a little bit of practice, it takes only a few weeks before you'll begin to see a major improvement in your posture.

Tips and Tricks

There's more to upholding great posture than just standing up straight all the time. Throughout the day, there are certain things that can easily bend you out of alignment if you're not careful. These easy-to-employ methods can keep your posture perfect, no matter where life tries to pull you.

Watch your chair time. Hours of sitting at a desk job can lead to back pain. So if you sit a lot, get up and walk around for five minutes out of every half hour of the day. Sitting for too long overstretches certain muscles while also placing stress on your discs and joints. Just getting up and moving around often can reduce that stress.

While you're out of your seat—stretch. Before returning to your seat (or immediately after getting up from it), loosen up your body several ways:

- Place your hands on the small of your back, then gently lean back as far as you comfortably can. Pause for three to five seconds, stand back up, and repeat.
- Raise your arms up above your head, then gently swoop forward and reach for your toes. (This works especially well when performed in front of your boss while saying out loud so everyone can hear, "Have you seen me do THIS?!?!!!")

When you're finally seated, sit the right way. Even if you're not constantly sitting all day, it's still important to maintain good posture whenever seated. Anytime you plop down, keep these posture pointers in mind:

- Face forward with your spine straight and shoulders back.
- You should feel your butt against the back of the chair.
- Instead of pressing your back into the chair to flatten it, stick a rolled-up shirt or towel between the chair and the curve just above your lower back.
- Avoid the lean. Shifting your bodyweight from side to side only creates undue stress.
- Don't cross your legs, and check your knees. Legs should be bent at a 90-degree angle (at least), with your knees either even with your hips or slightly higher. If they're not, lower your chair or place a box under your feet.
- Use the armrests, but position them correctly. They should be right at elbow height—if you have to lift, lower, or lean your arms forward to use them, adjust them.
- Monitor your monitor. If you are working in front of a computer screen, it should be at eye level and close enough so you don't have to squint. And if you're sitting right in front of your computer and still squinting, then forget the posture and go get your eyes checked.
- As you work, use the scroll bar often. Keeping whatever you're staring at at eye level will keep you from tilting your head down constantly all day long.

Use your neck—not your back—when looking up. Never arch your back if you need to stare up. Bending backward to see what's above you only places unnecessary pressure on the muscles of your lower back. Instead, bend at your neck (and adjust where you're standing if that's not a good enough view).

Use an earpiece—not your arm. Pinning the phone to your shoulder as you talk may be convenient in a pinch, but as any good telemarketer who uses one will tell you, it also tilts your head at an angle that overstretches the opposite side of your neck. Spare yourself the risk of pulling a muscle, which only validates that you spend way too much time on the phone, and buy an earpiece instead.

Adjust your seat whenever you're driving. Instead of angling the seat for comfort, pull the seat forward enough so your knees are positioned at a 90-degree angle—they should be even with (or higher than) your hips. As for the rest of you, adjust the headrest so that it's touching the back of your head, and take anything out of your pockets that could prevent you from sitting level.

Always be in good standing. Whenever you're stuck in one place, make sure your legs are aligned the right way. Your knees should be unlocked and your bodyweight should be evenly distributed across your feet rather than resting mostly on your heels.

Never fold—always bend. Anytime you need to pick something up such as a box, your suitcase, your kids, or the groceries, don't lean forward from your waist to reach down. Instead, stand directly in front of the object with your feet slightly wider than shoulder-width apart, then bend your knees so that your spine stays as straight as possible. Grab what you need and stand back up, keeping your back straight as you go.

Place posture reminders in places you tend to slouch. Enlist your kids (or a niece or nephew) to draw a few small pictures of someone standing straight and tall, then tape one at your desk, on your dashboard, anyplace where you tend to sit or stand improperly. To others, they will seem like proudly hung kid art. But every time you see them, they will be quick reminders to be aware of your posture.

Consider your footwear. Poorly fitted shoes, thick-soled shoes, and high heels all change the way you walk, shifting your body out of its natural alignment. Whenever possible, go barefoot. (Not in the office. I repeat: *not* in the office!) But when it's time to wear shoes, opt for anything with a thinner sole and low (to no) heel that lets your feet bend and flex.

Spend a third of your day the right way. How your body is positioned as you sleep is just as important as what it's doing when you're awake. Use only one pillow (but don't let your shoulders rest on it) and make sure your mattress is firm enough to support you.

- If you typically sleep on your back, tuck a pillow underneath your knees and a smaller one underneath your lower back for support.
- If you sleep on your side, stick a pillow between your knees to prevent your top knee from dropping down.
- If you sleep on your stomach, try not to. (Lying belly down places strain on your neck and back.) But if that's impossible, place a pillow underneath your hips.

CHANGE

#27

Substitute Sauces for Something Smarter

SIMPLY PUT . . . If you need to punch up the flavor of food, skip the sauce (which may contain extra calories, fat, and sugar) and use either a spice or a healthier sauce substitute instead.

My friend Marcy, bless her honest soul, always used to make fun of the food I ate. I guess you could call it food. She called it dirt. A fine array of kale, chia seeds, flaxseed, protein powder, Swiss chard, barley, bulgur, wheatgrass...Alright, I guess I can see how she could call it dirt. Clearly I ate more for nutrition and sustenance than taste and enjoyment.

I didn't worry about taste as long as it was healthy. Marcy, like most humans, didn't quite subscribe to the same food philosophy. So why was a boring culinary palate good enough for me? I just always assumed that drowning food in fattening sauces was the only way to add a little sex appeal. I knew no other option.

And then I met Stephanie. My partner in life. My lifesaver in the kitchen. My other option.

Steph loves food. She loves to make food out of other food. She loves interesting ingredients and subtle spices. And she opened my eyes to the wonderful world of taste. Oh, I still eat the same food—I just make it taste a little better so I eat a little more of it.

There are so many empty calories in the things we flood our food with, and it's far too easy to overdo using them once the drenching begins. But seasoning your foods with herbs and spices instead can strip away excess calories at every meal, adding plenty of flavor without the sodium, sugar, cholesterol, or fat most sauces and condiments come with.

DON'T STOP THERE...

Whichever herbs or spices you end up sprinkling on your foods is purely a matter of taste. But if you're staring at your wall o' spices thinking you have it all covered, there are a few things to know that could help you benefit from this Change even more. It's all about the planning.

How to Buy Them

- *If you have the patience, purchase them whole.* Whole spices last a lot longer than ground versions and taste fresher. If you go that route, you'll need either a spice grinder (a coffee grinder works too) or a mortar and pestle.
- *Don't go crazy buying them in bulk.* A little goes a long way with herbs and spices.
- *Use your nose and eyes.* When fresh, most spices are incredibly pungent and have a bright color. If a spice looks dull or smells musty, move on.

How to Store Them
If dry...

- *Store them the right way.* Always put them in airtight containers in a cool, dry, dark place. It may be convenient to have them hanging by your stove, but moisture, heat, and light can change their flavor.
- *Mark them with a date.* They may not spoil, but over time, herbs and spices become less potent and lose flavor. After you've had one for a year, it's time to toss it and start fresh.

- *What happens if the date rubs off?* Take a pinch and rub it between your fingers. If it has little to no smell, give it the heave-ho and get more.

If fresh...

- *Timing is everything.* Wait to buy them—or pull them from your herb garden—as close to the time you need to use them as possible.
- *Snip and soak them.* If storing them for a few days, cut the stems (when possible), place them in a glass of water (just like a flower), and refrigerate them. If you can't snip them, stick them in an open plastic bag in your crisper drawer.
- *Put them on ice.* If you won't be using them for a while, you can always freeze fresh herbs by washing them first, patting them dry, then removing the leaves and placing them in a freezer bag (either chopped or left whole).

How to Use Them
- *Start strong and stay small.* Stick with one strong herb or spice to start, then begin to add in one or two milder flavors if you need more. I learned this lesson the hard way when I thought it would be a good idea to use *all* the fresh spices in the house...at the same time...on the same piece of chicken. Even though it's a matter of taste, mixing two or more powerful herbs or spices—or too many herbs or spices in general—can easily overwhelm your food...and Stephanie.
- *Remember the rule: dried first and fresh last.* When cooking with herbs, add the dried kind early but save fresh herbs for the end or they can lose their flavor.
- *Dried is always stronger than fresh.* If a recipe calls for dried and you're using fresh, plan on using two to three times more fresh herbs.
- *Sprinkle in your palm—not over your food.* Shaking herbs or spices from a container onto anything steaming—a bubbling pot, a frying pan, even food that's warm on your plate—can put moisture in the container, causing dried spices to cake up.

A Few Must-Have Herbs and Spices to Try

Allspice (not to be confused with Old Spice)

The Taste: A mixture of cinnamon, cloves, and nutmeg—with a hint of pepper.

Often used in/with: Caribbean and Latin American dishes, although allspice works in stews, chili, and desserts such as cakes, cookies, and puddings.

Side benefit: The spice may aid digestion, relieve pain, and might have compounds that help reduce the growth of prostate cancer cells.[1]

Basil (sweet)

The Taste: Spicy-sweet with hints of licorice and clove.

Often used in/with: Italian dishes (especially meals involving tomatoes, pasta, chicken, fish, and shellfish), lamb, salads, soups, eggplant, and zucchini.

Side benefit: The fragrant herb also contains vitamin A, vitamin K, and lutein.

Cardamom

The Taste: Strong, fragrant, spicy, and sweet—merged into one!

Often used in/with: Indian and Scandinavian dishes, rice, pork, chicken, curry dishes, fruit, duck, lentils, peas, and squash.

Side benefit: It's rich in fiber, iron, and manganese, helps digestion, and may even fight cancer.[2]

Cayenne Pepper

The Taste: Hot…hot…hot!

Often used in/with: Mexican and Southwestern dishes, but also great used with soups, vegetables, fish, lean meats, eggs, and the obvious—chili.

Side benefit: The spice gets its heat from capsaicin, a compound found in many hot peppers that's been shown (among other perks) to relieve aches and pains, improve circulation, and boost your metabolism.

Celery Seed

The Taste: Ummm…like celery, only a smidge bitterer.

Often used in/with: Soups, stews, and burgers, or as a rub on steaks.

Side benefit: It's got calcium and iron, may lower blood pressure, and could help prevent arthritis.[3]

Chili Powder

The Taste: It's a mix of other spices (typically chili pepper, cumin, garlic, and oregano).

Often used in/with: Beans, rice, vegetables, stews, and soups, as a rub on chicken (or other meats), and the obvious—chili.

Side benefit: Because of its mix of spices, chili powder contains both vitamin A and vitamin C.

Cilantro

The Taste: Sage meets citrus!

Often used in/with: Asian, Latin American, and Mexican dishes, but also with poultry, fish, lamb, vegetables, pasta, salsas, salads, beans, rice, or shellfish.

Side benefit: It has fair amounts of both vitamin A and vitamin K.

Cinnamon

The Taste: You *really* don't know?

Often used in/with: Mexican and Greek dishes, desserts, coffee, oatmeal, toast, pork, carrots, fruit, cottage cheese, yogurt, sweet potatoes, and squash.

Side benefit: Extremely high in antioxidants compared to other spices (it's rich in calcium, iron, and manganese), it's also been shown to lower blood sugar and reduce inflammation.[4]

Coriander

The Taste: Toasted citrus that's mildly spicy.

Often used in/with: Curries, meat and seafood dishes, burgers, fish, shellfish, soups, stews, and many baked goods.

Side benefit: Coriander may help lower your blood sugar and cholesterol.

Cumin

The Taste: Nutty and mildly bitter.

Often used in/with: African, Indian, Middle Eastern, and Moroccan dishes, beans, rice, chili, stews, soups, vegetables, poultry, lamb, and fish dishes.

Side benefit: It may help with killing bacteria, controlling your blood pressure, and aiding digestion.[5,6,7]

Curry Powder

The Taste: This tangy spice is typically a blend of a variety of different spices, including cardamom, coriander, cumin, nutmeg, and turmeric— just to name a few.

Often used in/with: Indian or Southeast Asian dishes, meat, chicken, fish, rice, lamb, tomatoes, tofu, soups, and baked potatoes.

Side benefit: Although it depends on what mixture of spices is used, its multi-spice combo contains an array of antioxidants that could help minimize inflammation and aid digestion.

Dill

The Taste: A subtle mix of anise, celery, parsley, and lemon.

Often used in/with: Seafood, chicken, breads, soups, rice, pasta, vegetables (especially potatoes, cucumbers, and beets), egg dishes, and as a rub.

Side benefit: Dill has vitamin A, vitamin C, and quercetin, a flavonoid that helps reduce inflammation.[8]

Fennel

The Taste: Just like licorice (peppery and sweet).

Often used in/with: Italian dishes, sausage, fish, pork, pasta, and vegetables (especially beets and squash).

Side benefit: High in vitamin C, fennel has been shown to help with heartburn and is a natural appetite suppressant.

Garlic

The Taste: Again…you really don't know?!

Often used in/with: Lean meats, fish, poultry, soups, salads, and vegetables.

Side benefit: What doesn't it do? From boosting your immune system to fighting cancer, one of its compounds (allicin) has also been shown to lower your risk of heart disease and stroke.[9]

Ginger

The Taste: Slightly citrusy, but spicy-sweet.

Often used in/with: Asian, Indian, and Middle Eastern dishes, rice, meat, poultry, fish, soups, vegetables (especially carrots and squash), desserts, and oatmeal.

Side benefit: It eases your digestive system, prevents nausea, helps the absorption of essential nutrients, and it even has an anti-inflammatory effect.

Nutmeg

The Taste: Sweet and nutty.

Often used in/with: Indian and Middle Eastern dishes, veal, fish, chicken, vegetables (especially broccoli, cabbage, cauliflower, and spinach), milk- or cream-based dishes.

Side benefit: The essential oils found in nutmeg have been shown to have anti-inflammatory properties.

Oregano

The Taste: It's that smell wafting in every pizza place you've ever been to.

Often used in/with: Any Italian and Greek cuisine, meats, poultry, stews, salads, pizza, vegetables, and any tomato-, egg-, or cheese-based dish.

Side benefit: This common spice is thought to protect against cancer, reduce inflammation, and kill bad bacteria.[10,11]

Paprika

The Taste: Rich and smoky—although some types can have a little heat, ranging from mild to hot.

Often used in/with: Hungarian, German, and Spanish dishes, seafood, vegetables, goulash, eggs, soups, stews, rice, and as a rub.

Side benefit: Paprika contains vitamins A and E, as well as capsaicin, which helps rev up your metabolism.

Rosemary

The Taste: A fragrant lemony-pine flavor.

Often used in/with: Any meat, chicken, or fish dish (especially grilled), omelets, roasted or mashed potatoes, and most vegetables (particularly peas and mushrooms).

Side benefit: Not only might the herb improve your memory,[12] but it's believed to have antibacterial and antioxidant properties as well.

Sage

The Taste: Bitter and woody.

Often used in/with: Seafood, poultry, pork, soups and stews, vegetables, and baked goods.

Side benefit: It's great for your digestion and could help with memory and lowering cholesterol.

Tarragon

The Taste: Licorice.

Often used in/with: Egg and cheese dishes, tomato dishes, soups and stews, chicken, veal, fish, shellfish, meats, vegetables (especially asparagus, carrots, green beans, and mushrooms).

Side benefit: The tasty sprig has plenty of antioxidants and iron.

Thyme

The Taste: Mildly minty and lemony.

Often used in/with: Cheeses, egg or bean dishes, vegetables (especially eggplant, mushrooms, or summer squash), stews, soups, fish, chicken, shellfish, or rubbed on beef, pork, or lamb.

Side benefit: Plenty of vitamins and minerals, and one of the oils in the herb (thymol) is a strong antioxidant that could improve brain health.[13]

Turmeric

The Taste: Pungent and bitter.

Often used with: Indian and Moroccan dishes, meats, poultry, lamb, curries, stews, rice, salads, dips, and vegetables.

Side benefit: The mustard-yellow spice has been shown to have pain-relieving and anti-inflammatory properties and could help reduce memory loss in individuals with Alzheimer's disease.[14]

Tips and Tricks

If spices aren't cutting it for you and texture is what you crave, you do have a few options at your disposal that can still cut calories—without losing a bit of flavor.

Barbecue sauce: Most are sugar-laden and pile on calories that can go into the triple digits per serving. Instead, marinade your meat in a mix of low-sodium soy sauce and minced garlic for at least an hour, or try horseradish sauce, which can add some kick without the calories and sugar.

Ketchup: It may be made from tomatoes, but every tablespoon of the red staple is also loaded with sugar (4 grams' worth) and calories (on average, about 20)—and whoever pours out only one tablespoon's worth?! Seriously!

Instead, try a thin layer of sun-dried tomato hummus, salsa, or an actual slice of tomato. Or grab the bottle of yellow mustard right next to the ketchup (it's free of fat and sugar and has practically no calories).

Mayonnaise: Packed with preservatives and sugar, one tablespoon of the real stuff has about 90 calories and around 10 grams of fat. (The same spoonful of the light kind can still weigh in between 35 and 50 calories and 3.5–5 grams of fat—and even the fat-free kind has more than 10 calories a tablespoon.)

A few better options? Spread on some hummus, blend an avocado—it creates a similar texture and it's heart-healthy—or mix up a little Greek yogurt with a splash of lemon juice, a little mustard, and some pepper.

Ranch dressing: That delicious taste is usually an unhealthy combo of mayonnaise and sour cream. A better option: Stick with black bean dip, some hummus, plain yogurt flavored with a few spices (such as dill, garlic, and rosemary), or mix up some Dijon mustard, Parmesan cheese, and balsamic vinegar.

Salad dressing: Best of luck finding one that doesn't have fat, sugar, or soybean oil. Your best bet is to use olive oil or vinegar instead, or just make your own: Mix some lemon juice and a little olive oil, add salt and pepper, shake well—and voilà!

Spaghetti sauce: Sure, it's delicious, but most jarred versions have loads of sugar. Make it yourself or go with chopped tomatoes, fresh basil, and a hint of olive oil instead.

Tartar sauce: That fishy classic is just mayonnaise with a few things like parsley, chives, or capers thrown in. If your fish needs some flavor, try some pureed steamed veggies or Greek yogurt, or marinate your fish for at least three hours in a mix of soy sauce, vinegar, lime or lemon juice, a hint of olive oil, and a few spices and herbs.

#28

Drop One Stressful Thing in Your Life

SIMPLY PUT ... I want you to take a good, hard look at all of the things you're juggling/managing/stressing about in your life. Then, either drop one or find a smarter, more effective way to manage it.

Stress is tangible. You can feel it, you can see it, and you can smell and taste it. It visibly sits on you throughout every minute of every day, which should explain the tight shoulders, hunched back, and raging headaches.

Stress influences the choices you make, it affects the way you experience things, and it even impacts your relationships with others. But what's most concerning is what it's doing to your health. When you look at all of the horrible things we do to our bodies, stress is right up there. It's linked to every major illness you can think of, including cancer, depression, and heart disease. And we're all victims to it.

There is stress in my life. There is stress in your life. But there's got to be at least one thing on your stress plate right now that really doesn't need to be there. Maybe you're worrying about something that's not your problem. Are you still stewing about something that happened years ago?

If you're not sure what it might be, just ask your friends or family what they think you worry about more than you should. Trust me—it will be the one thing that keeps coming up. The same thing that probably comes up anytime someone close to you has said, "Hey, don't worry about it—that's not your problem."

Guess what? That's the one you can probably let go.

DON'T STOP THERE...

Thanks to the Changes you've already introduced into your life through this book (exercising more, eating better, and managing your time more efficiently to get things done, for example), you've already begun reducing a great deal of the stress in your life. But if you're still holding on to more (and we're all guilty of it), it could be keeping you from breaking out of your rut.

I can't tell you to *completely* avoid or drop everything that stresses you out because that's unrealistic. In many ways, life is the ultimate stress test. Between work, family, friends, dating, diets, and money, it's all around us. But while we can't rid ourselves of it entirely, we can learn to control how we react and respond to it.

Face each stressor head–on. People ask me all the time: "How do you juggle everything—kids, job, travel, working out, training, family—and still stay sane?" First I casually mention that sanity is overrated. Then I explain I have a good working relationship with stress, and so should you. In other words: Dear Stress, Let's break up, but can we remain friends?

The biggest mistake people make is ignoring whatever's stressing them out in the first place. So as each new stressor plops in your lap, you pretend that it's not there invading your personal space. Don't ignore it—acknowledge it. Stare it down. Look at its existence and immediately start planning a way to deal with it. The sooner you take it on, the less time you'll spend concerned about it.

Always be in the present. We've become a world of multitaskers. But if you're sitting down in a work meeting and your brain is trying to figure out who is going to watch your sixteen-month-old this weekend, what you're making for dinner tonight, how you're going to have time to work out tomorrow, and what you're going to say in your speech at Marcy's wedding *next* October, you'll end up drowning in your own stressful misery. (Go with a poem, by the way—they're always showstoppers at weddings.)

Instead, one trick that works for me to minimize stress is to focus only on whatever is on my plate at that very moment—and that's it. I surprise people when I suggest this because they assume I'm constantly doing a million things at once. It's not that I don't get a million things done—it's just that I give each of those million things their due (and it's more like three million, to be honest).

For me, that's the only way I've ever been able to manage everything. If I'm sitting in a meeting, that's the only thing that I'm focused on. If I'm at home with my daughters, telling them about a new variation on the push-up (relax, I'm just kidding), then that's all that I'm focused on. If you forget about trying to do everything at once—and just do one thing at a time—you'll be surprised how everything seems to work out with less stress.

Give 100 percent to that one thing in front of you. Once you've pinpointed whatever is causing you stress, give it all the attention it deserves. Don't half-ass it. Deal with it completely; otherwise it remains on your stress plate, just in a different form. If you have ten bills to pay, sit down and pay them all. Don't pay a few now and put some in your bag to do tomorrow when you get to work. Deal with it. Cross if off your list. Move on.

By not taking advantage of the time you have, you walk away with regret. You walk away saying, "Ugh! I didn't spend enough time on that" or "I didn't put my best foot forward." But if you step away from a stressful situation knowing you did your best, you'll walk away from it carrying less guilt and have more energy to tackle it the next time.

Tips and Tricks

When stress strikes, it's good to have a few other things up your sleeve besides listening to music or meditating to melt it all away. (Both are sound options for calming yourself down though.) Now, before you reject the following as silly or ridiculous or incapable of working, give them a try.

Find a four-legged friend. Grab a dog, cat, or any other animal you're not allergic to that won't bite or poop on you, and spend some time petting it. Research has shown that petting an animal may not only help to lower your blood pressure, it also decreases the amount of the stress hormone cortisol and increases the release of feel-good endorphins such as serotonin and oxytocin.

Show your partner some love. Hugging, kissing, sex—even just holding your partner's hand—has been shown to lower blood pressure, release oxytocin, and drive down cortisol.

Double up on your outdoor time. Walking 10,000 steps *should* be getting you outside more, but if the only times you find yourself exposed to fresh air are the brief moments between leaving your car and going into whatever building you drove it to, then get outside already. Not only does natural light increase your body's levels of serotonin, but nature has a way of helping your brain instantly unwind.

Rotate a few stress-fighting foods into your diet. Some fruits, vegetables, and meats contain certain nutrients that have not only been shown to reduce symptoms that can occur with stress, but may even lower your stress levels altogether. The next time you're preparing a meal or snack, try a few of the following:

- *Asparagus (and broccoli):* Both have high levels of folic acid, a mood-enhancing nutrient that prevents depression and stabilizes your mood.
- *Avocados:* Rich in potassium and monounsaturated fats—both of which help to lower your blood pressure—they're also loaded with B vitamins, which combat stress as well.
- *Fatty fish:* Halibut, salmon, and tuna are all high in omega-3 fatty acids, great for boosting serotonin and reducing the level of cortisol in your system. Those fatty acids also contain DHA (docosahexaenoic acid), which nourishes your brain so it functions more efficiently—and you have an easier time managing your stress.
- *Nuts and seeds:* A great source of stress-fighting omega-3 fatty acids, some (like cashews and sunflower seeds) also contain the amino acid L-tryptophan, which boosts the release of serotonin.
- *Oatmeal:* Not only is this complex carbohydrate great for leaving you feeling fuller longer, it's also been shown to increase serotonin production and contains magnesium, a mineral shown to regulate cortisol and create a feeling of well-being in most people.
- *Spinach:* The vegetable has a calming effect on many people due to providing nearly 40 percent of the recommended daily allowance of magnesium.

- *Turkey:* There's a reason you feel sleepy after eating this bird. It's teeming with tryptophan. But if your access to the bird only happens around the holidays, a glass of milk has plenty of tryptophan in it too.
- *Vitamin C–rich foods:* Berries, citrus fruits, tomatoes, broccoli, peppers, kale—any food that's fortified with vitamin C helps you combat stress by lowering cortisol.

Make what's around you smell nicer. Certain scents have been shown to relieve stress, so try a few of the tried-and-true aromas, like vanilla, lavender, rosemary, chamomile, cypress, pizza, or even baby powder. (Sorry about that. Pizza always tries to squeeze itself into the mix in my world.)

Leave work at the office—and at your hamper. The minute you get home from work or anyplace that requires you to wear something less relaxing, slip into something more comfortable (said in a sexy voice). Just the act of changing can make you feel as if you're leaving whatever problems you had throughout the day behind.

Call the funniest friend you know. There's a reason we all could use a good laugh. Laughter elevates the release of endorphins and lowers stress hormones such as cortisol and epinephrine. So go ahead. Call the one person who you know will crack you up. (My number is 917-48...)

Set your clock fifteen minutes fast. A great deal of stress doesn't come from the things we have to do—it's waiting until the last minute to do them that causes undue stress. Budgeting enough time to your tasks can strip away stress before it ever occurs.

Find a chore that's mindless but still challenging. Take on a project that requires time and a lot of physical effort but isn't something that requires much thought or needs to be done right away. Whether it's yard work, cleaning out a closet, or folding laundry, don't discount the power of letting your brain turn off and your body take over to shed stress.

The "So You Know" Science

Even if you take great pride in piling on stress to prove you can handle anything, know that stress is actually the one handling you.

Whenever you're stressed out, your adrenal glands on top of your kidneys secrete cortisol. This fight-or-flight hormone is meant to help your body respond to stress by (among other things) raising your blood pressure and blood sugar, so you have the energy to either fight what's in front of you or run like hell. But when you're always stressed, that stream of cortisol never stops, which becomes detrimental to your body.

The short-term effects can range from insomnia and having a harder time concentrating to experiencing a lower libido, headaches, high blood pressure, chronic pain, fatigue, and an upset stomach. Studies have even associated cortisol with our bodies accumulating belly fat and developing cravings for fat-laden and sugary foods.

But the long-term effects are far worse. Because stress can affect nearly every function within your body, it's a major contributor to heart disease, weight gain, depression, fertility issues, acne and eczema, ulcers, and arthritis.

#29

Perform a 60-Minute Workout 3X a Week

SIMPLY PUT...Starting today, I want you to do some form of a 60-minute full-body strength-training workout three times a week. You'll stop doing the workout from Change #24 (the 45-minute workout I showed you), but you'll continue to walk 10,000 steps each day.

Let's crunch some numbers and play with a little perspective here: A 60-minute workout is only 4 percent of your day. Four percent is nothing!! And I'm only asking you to do that three days a week. That's 180 minutes, or exactly 1.786 percent of your entire week. And if you look around at some of the other nonproductive things we waste just under 2 percent of our time doing weekly—sitting in meetings, online shopping, texting, posting, friending—exercising for that *short* a time has way more to offer you.

Praise the Pyramid

Remember I told you about my friend Marni who lost twenty pounds in eight months after I switched her old workout to a pyramid routine (ten exercises done in a row that decrease in repetitions while increasing in difficulty)? Well, now it's your turn—and here's why:

When I was younger—single, carefree, and childless, with no responsibilities or demands on my time—I would fill up my social calendar with gym classes every night. Cycling, boot camp, kickboxing, Pilates, yoga, kettlebells, step, abs—you name it and I did it. (You'll be surprised to know I was single a lot during that stretch!)

Some of those classes had staying power, like cycling and boot camps, while others…well, didn't. I still have flashbacks of a ridiculous stretch band class where we tied exercise bands to our ankles and walked across the floor. Those cheap bands were snapping apart all over the place! We all limped out of class afterward with band marks all over our legs!!!

The point is that I had time to do it all—even the stuff that wasted my time.

And then life happened. Between my job, family obligations, traveling, social engagements—you know, grown-up stuff—my free nights filled up fast. I no longer had the time to venture out every night (or any night) to try new classes, test out new equipment, or visit little boutique gyms. But my appetite for a great sweat was still there.

So I put together a workout that could be done in ten-minute chunks of time. A workout that required no equipment, space, gym, instructor, or money to do it—so I had no excuse *not* to do it. A routine that hit every muscle group, combined cardiovascular training and strength training, and, because it could be repeated over and over again without boredom setting in, I could use it whether I only had ten minutes to give—or twenty, thirty, forty, fifty, or sixty minutes.

It's called a pyramid workout, where you do ten exercises back-to-back for ten minutes. The first exercise you'll do for 100 reps, followed by 90, 80, 70, and so on (down to 10 reps). Even though you'll do each exercise for ten less reps as you go, the order of the exercises is from easiest to hardest—so believe me when I tell you, doing the last exercise for 10 reps will be *just* as demanding as doing the first one for 100 reps.

I use pyramids all the time now, and they've become the backbone behind how I stay in "on-air" shape year-round. If I only have twenty minutes to spare because of my hectic schedule, I'll try to get through two full pyramids without stopping. On days when I have more time, I'll aim for a full six in an hour.

The Game Plan: These two final workouts should only take you about ten minutes each to complete, using exercises you're already familiar with from previous chapters (and a few new ones I think you'll love). You'll run through all ten exercises without resting. After you've completed a pyramid, you'll rest for only one minute, then repeat the pyramid.

Once you're finished:

- You can repeat the pyramid five more times (for a total of six pyramids) to achieve a 60-minute workout.
- If you're not quite there yet physically, you can repeat the pyramid two, three, or four more times for a full 30-, 40-, or 50-minute workout (then work your way up until you can complete six pyramids).

Just like every other workout you've pulled off up until now, there are those few rules you must follow to make sure your muscles are ready for what's ahead—and get enough of a break between workouts:

- Before each workout, do a quick five-minute warm-up.
- Take one day off between sessions to let your muscles rest and recover.

THE WORKOUTS

Start with Level One first. Trust me, you won't grow bored with it—and the day you do, look down, because you'll be in incredible shape. But if you're looking for even more of a challenge, move on to Level Two when you feel you're ready.

BTW, no one knows your muscles better than you do, so I'm letting you know this: You're not limited to these two pyramids. In fact, I encourage you to create your own, once you get the hang of these. So long as you take ten cardio and strength exercises that collectively work all your major muscle groups, then place them in order of difficulty from easiest to hardest, the sky's the limit. Just make sure that anything you create is as taxing as the workouts in this chapter.

Pyramid 1 (Level One)

(Do this circuit 1 time)

- 100 jogs in place
- 90 hip raises
- 80 jumping jacks
- 70 one-legged reverse claps standing on your left leg, then 70 standing on your right leg
- 60 pikes
- 50 wall push-offs
- 40 crab kicks (left leg, right leg = 1 rep)
- 30 squats
- 20 plank toe lifts
- 10 slow mountain climbers

Pyramid 2 (Level Two)

(Do this circuit 1 time)

- 100 jumping jacks (To make the move even more intense, try holding a pair of 1-, 2-, or 3-pound hand weights.)
- 90 jogs in place
- 80 quad drops
- 70 butt kickers
- 60 pikes
- 50 squats
- 40 push-ups on your knees
- 30 toy soldiers
- 20 slow mountain climbers
- 10 high squat jumps

THE EXERCISES

Pyramid 1

Jogs in Place (see page 71)

Hip Raises (see page 32)

Jumping Jacks (see page 72)

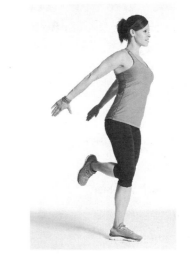

One-Legged Reverse Claps

SETUP: Stand straight with your arms extended behind you, palms facing each other. Raise your right foot behind you so that you're balancing on your left foot.

THE MOTION: Keeping your arms straight (or as straight as possible because of the angle), quickly move your arms in and out toward each other as if you were applauding, but don't let your hands touch each other. Instead, try to get them as close as possible without touching. Bringing your arms in and pulling them out equals 1 rep. Do the required number of reps, then switch positions—this time balancing on your right foot only—and repeat.

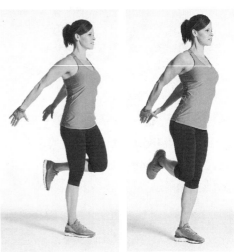

Note: The higher you can raise your arms as you go, the more you'll work the back of your arms—but don't hunch over or look down.

Pikes (see page 33)

Wall Push-offs (see page 39)

Crab Kicks (see page 31)

Squats (see page 36)

Plank Toe Lifts

SETUP: Get in a push-up position— legs extended behind you, feet together with your weight on your toes. Bend your arms and rest on your forearms. (Your body should be in a straight line from your head to your heels.)

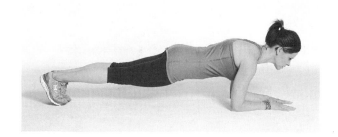

THE MOTION: Keeping yourself in the plank position, lift your right foot off the ground a few inches, then lower it back down. Repeat the same movement with your left foot—that's 1 rep.

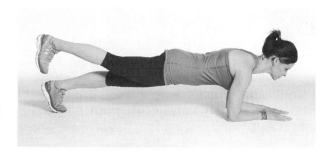

Slow Mountain Climbers (see page 34)

Pyramid 2

Jumping Jacks (see page 72)

Jogs in Place (see page 71)

Quad Drops (see page 76)

Butt Kickers (see page 119)

Pikes (see page 33)

Squats (see page 36)

Kneeling Push-ups (see page 40)

Toy Soldiers (see page 37)

Slow Mountain Climbers (see page 34)

High Squat Jumps

THE MOTION: Quickly squat down until your thighs are almost parallel to the floor, then jump straight up as high as possible, bringing your arms back as far as you comfortably can. As you land, gently bend your knees and return to a squat position (arms out in front of you) and repeat.

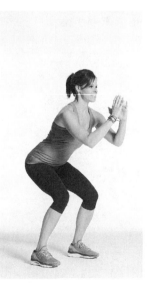
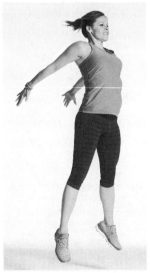

Tips and Tricks

You can use any of the tips and tricks I suggested with the 45-minute workout you're no longer performing. But now that you're involved with a full 60-minute routine, I want you to have even more to draw from.

Try working out on the same days each week. The more loosely and casually planned your workouts are, the more convenient it can be to cancel them. Instead, pick specific days of the week and block out that hour as if it's an important meeting. You'll be less inclined to miss it if you pencil it in first and then plan the rest of your day around it.

Breathe in and breathe out. Sounds easy, right? You've been doing it literally all your life. But a lot of people make the mistake of holding their breath at certain spots when they exercise. Don't do that: It can raise your blood pressure and deprive you of the oxygen your body needs for energy. As you go, just breathe naturally and as deeply as you can with each breath.

Take your pulse before breakfast. When it comes to pushing your body *too much* from exercise, everyone's different. But I want to be sure you're not overtraining, which can cause fatigue, moodiness, persistent muscular soreness, and sleep problems.

One way to monitor yourself is by taking your pulse first thing in the morning. Once you have that number, just look for any changes by checking your pulse the morning after your workouts. If it's more than eight to ten beats per minute above normal, your body may need a rest day to recuperate.

Sip according to what you sweat. Sixty minutes is a long time, so to make sure you're replacing the water you'll be sweating out, you could weigh yourself right before you begin your workout. After you're finished, weigh yourself again—and no, that difference on the scale isn't fat you've burned off like some trainers might have you believe (it's just water). For every pound you've lost, drink around a pint (sixteen ounces) of water and you'll be back to normal.

The "So You Know" Science

If 180 minutes still sounds like a lot of time to devote each week to exercise to have a stronger heart, build lean muscles, and torch excess body fat, would you do it if I told you it might keep you alive five years longer?

That's right—research published in the *American Journal of Preventive Medicine*[1] discovered that doing some form of exercise for at least 150 minutes a week could extend your life by as much as five years. Part of that might be due to the fact that regular exercise has been proven to lower your risk of many chronic diseases and medical conditions (such as cancer, diabetes, and hypertension).

Today show Tested

My friend Natalie Morales is a runner. Not just an *"Oh, it's a nice day out so I think I'll go for a cute little jog in the park"* type of runner. She is a multiple marathon–running machine.

I, on the other hand, am not a runner. A high school sports injury (short for "I hurt my knee playing volleyball," but *sports injury* sounds fancier) forced me to tweak my workout routine to substitute running—which places a lot of pressure on your knees—with other types of cardio. In my case: the pyramid.

So when I was talking to Natalie about working out and invited her to do a pyramid with me, I'm sure a 10-minute workout sounded adorable, especially to a marathon runner who's used to running for hours. But instead of convincing her, I just asked her to join me. Up for any challenge, Nat agreed.

It didn't take long for her to realize this wasn't a throwaway workout. The two of us sweated and grunted and muscled our way through it. Truth be told, I did build a particularly hard pyramid that morning. But it was the same concept (a good mix of cardio and strength moves with no breaks in between) that kept her motivated. And she quickly learned that it's not always how many minutes you work out but what you pour into those minutes that counts.

And we poured everything into those ten minutes.

For a runner, this gave Natalie a new creative and challenging workout to add to her mix. And because she doesn't always have time to go out for a twenty-seven-hour run (don't laugh, she could probably do it), this was the perfect way to fit a workout into any amount of time she has.

After finishing up the last exercise of the pyramid, I asked her if she wanted to join me for five more just like it to round out the hour. Let's just say we're still "coordinating" schedules to make that happen.

CHANGE #30

It's You—So Go Look in the Mirror Already!

So, you've arrived at the very last chapter...the thirtieth Change. Welcome, and congratulations. You've taken a small chunk of time out of your long, busy life to commit to *you*. Doesn't that feel good? So now, you ask, what next?

Whether you're here because you've just begun the Changes, completed them all, or are somewhere in between, you should be proud of yourself for taking back control of your life.

If, however, you haven't even started yet, what are you waiting for? (And please don't say Monday. That's a lot of pressure to put on the poor day.) The truth is, you will never be 100 percent ready to change—ever. So don't wait for the perfect day of the perfect month, because it'll never come. As it turns out, the perfect time is actually right this second—it's literally right now.

For the rest of you, who've been following all twenty-nine Changes, I want you to know something: This is not the end, it's only the beginning. There's no finish line. The goal was to give you thirty Changes that jump-started your health from *"I don't know where to start"* to *"Look at me! I feel great. I'm moving great. I'm eating great. Let's keep going!"*

So now, I hand over the reins to you.

You understand what you have to do to stay in shape—not because you've read about it but because you've *done* it.

This journey was never about doing this *for* you, it was always about doing it *with* you. The day I started writing this book, I was staring at myself in the mirror a few weeks after giving birth to my second daughter. I knew that I couldn't just write about change *for* you, I had to dive in, get dirty, and do each of the Changes, one by one, right alongside you. I had to prove to myself that every single word in this book was part of my own overall plan to lose that weight, get back in shape again, and stay in love with the person looking back at me in the mirror.

So when you tell me it's hard to start, I know— I was there. When you tell me you have tough days when carbs are calling out to you from across the kitchen, I know—I was there. When you tell me there are times when you absolutely do not want to work out, when the gym seems less appealing than a bikini wax, I completely hear you (and I apologize for the analogy). But my options were simple:

Either I quit and went all the way back to square one (the loneliest shape), or I pushed through and lived in discomfort for a few seconds to reap many rewards. I chose option B. I kept going, much like you can and you will. And now I'm here, sharing my journey with you in small pieces.

So I guess what I'm saying is, after twenty-nine Changes that have guided you from THEN to NOW, the last one is very simple and yet the most important one. The last Change (drumroll please)...is YOU.

You're the one who decides what you eat, when you work out, where you find time to relax, why you keep quitting, and how you'll reengage for good.

So I will leave you with this last piece of advice: *Simply put, whenever you feel scared, doubtful, insecure, confused, weak, or fragile—whenever you want to quit, stop, cheat, cry, beg, or break—I want you to say to yourself, "I can and I will."*

Say it to the person next to you.

Say it as a whisper.

Say it as a prayer.

Say it in Spanish.

I don't care. Just say it.

"I can and I will."

Final actual phone conversation with my parents

ME: Hey, guys. What are you doing?

MOM: Just cleaning up from dinner. Thinking of taking a walk now that it's warmer out.

ME: Nice! What did you have for dinner?

MOM: We grilled salmon with broccoli and a big salad. And some pineapple for dessert.

ME: Wow, Mom, that's great!

MOM: And now we're going for a walk.

ME: Yeah, you just mentioned that.

MOM: All those times you thought we weren't listening to all your advice, we actually were. And now we're eating better and starting to exercise with the walking.

ME: Again with the walking. You feel good?

MOM: Your father lost eight pounds and I lost five. Here, say hello.

DAD: Hey, honey...Did your mom tell you we're walking now?

ME: Briefly.

DAD: We love the changes we've made thanks to you.

ME: I'm curious. What changes?

DAD: Drink water, don't eat pasta after six, and keep a diary.

ME: A *food* diary. Not a regular diary. Keep a **food** diary. Anyway, go for your walk. I'll talk to you later. Where are you going, by the way?

DAD: Oh, they're having a cheese *and* cheesecake festival in town tonight. Who knew they paired together?!?

(*Dead silence*)

ME: I give up.

Acknowledgments

My parents, Sheila and Bennett: You encouraged every adventure, and softened every fall. My tireless heroes.

My brother, Michael, and my sister-in-law Jill: Michael, my first friend. I always admired that you could quote *Seinfeld* lines with me all day and then go operate all night. Thankfully you're a doctor.

The Today **show:** For saying yes to all my crazy fitness ideas and helping me build a platform to get our audience back in shape.

Lester Holt: My gym buddy, office neighbor, and Jamaican brother...sort of.

My agent, Scott Wachs: For making me see what my future could/should/will look like.

Andy McNicol: For pushing my baby through to publication. And by baby, I mean book idea.

Marni Bernstein: My best friend. My first client. My confidence, even during the rough patches. You believed in me before I believed in me.

Marcy Olin: Thank you for all the life lessons you taught/showed me. You didn't know it, but I listened to every single one.

My friends who have supported, partaken in, produced, or encouraged my calorie-blasting lifestyle: Marcy Olin, Michelle Sorscher, Josh Weiner, Josh Glatt, Saskia Fisher, Jeff Rossen, Jarred Snyder, Joel Harper, Carol Snyder, Alisa Mall, the guy in my gym who always lets me use the medicine ball, Lindsay Grubb,

Erica Hill, Dylan Dreyer, Natalie Morales, and Sam Wender, producer, friend, right hand, left hand...thank you.

Myatt Murphy: My brain. Honestly. None of this would have gotten written, shot, organized, or finished without you.

My publishing team at Hachette: Liz Connor, Nick Small, Amanda Pritzker, Karen Murgolo, Yasmin Mathew, Morgan Hedden, Brittany Hamblin, and last but not least, my editor, Sarah Pelz. You loved my pitch from our very first meeting and maintained that rare and refreshing zeal throughout this whole process—you are a gem in a very busy literary world.

Everyone that was a part of my cover and interior shoot: Esteban Aladro, Nate Mumford, Kathy Kalafut, and especially Beth Bischoff—you made me come alive through your lens. And a big hair 'n makeup thank you to Wilfredo Sanchez and Deborah Bell. I'd be frizzy-haired and pale without you.

Finally, those who bullied me in school because I didn't fit in: Turns out, not fitting in just forced me to stand out.

Notes

CHANGE #5

1. "Why Strength Training?," Centers for Disease Control and Prevention, accessed May 22, 2015, http://www.cdc.gov/physicalactivity/growingstronger/why/.

CHANGE #8

1. Jessié M. Gutierres et al., "Neuroprotective Effect of Anthocyanins on Acetyl-cholinesterase Activity and Attenuation of Scopolamine-Induced Amnesia in Rats," *International Journal of Developmental Neuroscience* 33 (April 2014): 88–97, doi:10.1016/j.ijdevneu.2013.12.006.

2. Kendra J. Royston and Trygve O. Tollefsbol, "The Epigenetic Impact of Cruciferous Vegetables on Cancer Prevention," *Current Pharmacology Reports* 1, no. 1 (February 2015): 46–51, doi:10.1007/s40495-014-0003-9.

3. Rose K. Davidson et al., "Sulforaphane Represses Matrix-Degrading Proteases and Protects Cartilage from Destruction in Vitro and in Vivo," *Arthritis and Rheumatism* 65, no. 12 (December 2013): 3130–40, doi:10.1002/art.38133.

4. "Beta-Carotene," Medline Plus, U.S. National Library of Medicine, last reviewed February 13, 2015, http://www.nlm.nih.gov/medlineplus/druginfo/natural/999.html.

5. "Cruciferous Vegetables and Cancer Prevention," National Cancer Institute at the National Institutes of Health, reviewed June 7, 2012, http://www.cancer.gov/cancertopics/causes-prevention/risk/diet/cruciferous-vegetables-fact-sheet.

6. Anette Karlsen et al., "Anthocyanins Inhibit Nuclear Factor-kappaB Activation in Monocytes and Reduce Plasma Concentrations of Pro-inflammatory Mediators in Healthy Adults," *Journal of Nutrition* 137, no. 8 (August 2007): 1951–54.

7. Jouni Karppi, "Serum Lycopene Decreases the Risk of Stroke in Men: A Population-Based Follow-Up Study," *Neurology* 79, no. 15 (October 9, 2012): 1540–47, doi:10.1212/WNL.0b013e31826e26a6.

8. "Protective Effects of Lycopene Against Ultraviolet B-Induced Photodamage," *Nutr Cancer.* 2003;47(2):181-7.

9. O. Benavente-Garcia and J. Castillo, "Update on Uses and Properties of Citrus Flavonoids: New Findings in Anticancer, Cardiovascular, and Anti-inflammatory Activity," *Journal of Agricultural and Food Chemistry* 56, no. 15 (August 2008): 6185–205, doi:10.1021/jf8006568.

10. Guillaume Ruel et al., "Impact of Low-Calorie Cranberry Juice Consumption on Plasma HDL-Cholesterol Concentrations in Men," *British Journal of Nutrition* 96, no. 2 (August 2006): 357–64, doi:10.1079/BJN20061814.

11. Bridget D. Mathison et al., "Consumption of Cranberry Beverage Improved Endogenous Antioxidant Status and Protected Against Bacteria Adhesion in Healthy Humans: A Randomized Controlled Trial," *Nutrition Research* 34, no. 5 (May 2014): 420–27, doi:10.1016/j.nutres.2014.03.006.

12. Maneli Mozaffarieh, Stefan Sacu, and Andreas Wedrich, "The Role of the Carotenoids, Lutein and Zeaxanthin, in Protecting Against Age-Related Macular Degeneration: A Review Based on Controversial Evidence," *Nutrition Journal* 2, no. 20 (December 2003), doi:10.1186/1475-2891-2-20.

13. Arja T. Erkkilä and Alice H. Lichtenstein, "Fiber and Cardiovascular Disease Risk: How Strong Is the Evidence?," *Journal of Cardiovascular Nursing* 21, no. 1 (January/February 2006): 3–8, doi:10.1097/00005082-200601000-00003.

14. "Whole Grains and Fiber," American Heart Association, updated May 15, 2015, http://www.heart.org/HEARTORG/GettingHealthy/NutritionCenter/HealthyDiet-Goals/Whole-Grains-and-Fiber_UCM_303249_Article.jsp.

15. "Manganese," Medline Plus, U.S. National Library of Medicine, reviewed February 15, 2015, http://www.nlm.nih.gov/medlineplus/druginfo/natural/182.html.

16. R. Corder et al., "Oenology: Red Wine Procyanidins and Vascular Health," *Nature* 444 (November 2006): 566, doi:10.1038/444566a.

17. "Ellagic acid induces cell cycle arrest and apoptosis through TGF-β/Smad3 signaling pathway in human breast cancer MCF-7 cells." *Int J Oncol.* 2015 Apr;46(4):1730-8.

18. "Vitamin A," Medline Plus, U.S. National Library of Medicine, updated February 18, 2013, http://www.nlm.nih.gov/medlineplus/ency/article/002400.htm.

19. O. Sommerburg et al., "Fruits and Vegetables That Are Sources for Lutein and Zeaxanthin: The Macular Pigment in Human Eyes," *British Journal of Ophthalmology* 82, no. 8 (August 1998): 907–10, http://www.ncbi.nlm.nih.gov/pmc/articles/PMC1722697/.

20. "Lutein & Zeaxanthin," American Optometric Association, accessed May 22, 2015, http://www.aoa.org/patients-and-public/caring-for-your-vision/diet-and-nutrition/lutein?sso=y.

CHANGE #9

1. Nicolaas P. Pronk et al., "Reducing Occupational Sitting Time and Improving Worker Health: The Take-a-Stand Project, 2011," Centers for Disease Control and Prevention, *Preventing Chronic Disease* 9 (2012), doi:http://dx.doi.org/10.5888/pcd9.110323.

CHANGE #11

1. "ACE Study Finds Fitness Benefits of Wearing Casual Clothing to Work," American Council on Exercise, July 14, 2004, https://www.acefitness.org/about-ace/press-room/339/ace-study-finds-fitness-benefits-of-wearing-casual/.

CHANGE #13

1. "Increasing the Number of Chews before Swallowing Reduces Meal Size in Normal-Weight, Overweight, and Obese Adults," June 2014, Volume 114, Issue 6, 926–931.

CHANGE #23

1. Qing Yang, "Gain Weight by 'Going Diet?' Artificial Sweeteners and the Neurobiology of Sugar Cravings," *Yale Journal of Biology and Medicine* 83, no. 2 (June 2010): 101–8, http://www.ncbi.nlm.nih.gov/pmc/articles/PMC2892765/.

CHANGE #25

1. "WHO Calls on Countries to Reduce Sugars Intake Among Adults and Children," World Health Organization, March 4, 2015, http://www.who.int/mediacentre/news/releases/2015/sugar-guideline/en/.

2. "Frequently Asked Questions About Sugar," American Heart Association, updated May 19, 2014, http://www.heart.org/HEARTORG/GettingHealthy/NutritionCenter/HealthyEating/Frequently-Asked-Questions-About-Sugar_UCM_306725_Article.jsp.

CHANGE #27

1. Nagarajarao Shamaladevi, "Ericifolin: A Novel Antitumor Compound from Allspice That Silences Androgen Receptor in Prostate Cancer," *Carcinogenesis* 34, no. 8 (August 2013), doi:10.1093/carcin/bgt123.

2. Christine M. Kaefer and John A. Milner, "Herbs and Spices in Cancer Prevention and Treatment," in Iris F. F. Benzie and Sissi Wachtel-Galor, eds., *Herbal Medicine: Biomolecular and Clinical Aspects*, 2nd edition. (Boca Raton, FL: CRC Press, 2011), 361–82.

3. "Find a Vitamin or Supplement: Celery," WedMD, accessed May 22, 2015, http://www.webmd.com/vitamins-supplements/ingredientmono-882-celery.aspx?activeingredientid=882&activeingredientname=celery.

4. B. Qin, K. S. Panickar, and R. A. Anderson, "Cinnamon: Potential Role in the Prevention of Insulin Resistance, Metabolic Syndrome, and Type 2 Diabetes," *Journal of Diabetes Science and Technology* 4, no. 3 (May 2010): 685–93, http://www.ncbi.nlm.nih.gov/pubmed/20513336.

5. Tolou Allahghadri et al., "Antimicrobial Property, Antioxidant Capacity, and Cytotoxicity of Essential Oil from Cumin Produced in Iran," *Journal of Food Science* 75, no. 2 (March 2010): H54–61, doi:10.1111/j.1750-3841.2009.01467.x.

6. K. S. Muthamma Milan et al., "Enhancement of Digestive Enzymatic Activity by Cumin (*Cuminum cyminum* L.) and Role of Spent Cumin as a Bionutrient," *Food Chemistry* 110, no. 3 (October 2008): 678–83, doi:10.1016/j.foodchem.2008.02.062.

7. K. Platel and K. Srinivasan, "Digestive Stimulant Action of Spices: A Myth or Reality?," *Indian Journal of Medical Research* 119, no. 5 (May 2004): 167–79.

8. Yazdani B. Shaik et al., "Role of Quercetin (a Natural Herbal Compound) in Allergy and Inflammation," *Journal of Biological Regulators and Homeostatic Agents* 20, no. 3–4 (July-December 2006): 47–52.

9. "Garlic," National Center for Complementary and Integrative Health, updated April 2012, https://nccih.nih.gov/health/garlic/ataglance.htm.

10. I. Savini et al., "Origanum Vulgare Induces Apoptosis in Human Colon Cancer Caco2 Cells," *Nutrition and Cancer* 61, no. 3 (2009): 381–89, doi:10.1080/01635580802582769.

11. "Salutary Pizza Spice: Oregano Helps Against Inflammations," *ScienceDaily*, June 26, 2008, http://www.sciencedaily.com/releases/2008/06/080625093147.htm.

12. "Rosemary Aroma May Help You Remember to Do Things," *ScienceDaily*, April 9, 2013, www.sciencedaily.com/releases/2013/04/130409091104.htm.

13. K. A. Youdim and S. G. Deans, "Effect of Thyme Oil and Thymol Dietary Supplementation on the Antioxidant Status and Fatty Acid Composition of the Ageing Rat Brain," *British Journal of Nutrition* 83, no. 1 (January 2000): 87–93.

14. Shrikant Mishra and Kalpana Palanivelu, "The Effect of Curcumin (Turmeric) on Alzheimer's Disease: An Overview," *Annals of Indian Academy of Neurology* 11, no. 1 (January-March 2008): 13–19, doi:10.4103/0972-2327.40220.

CHANGE #29

1. Ian Janssen et al., "Years of Life Gained due to Leisure-Time Physical Activity in the U.S.," *American Journal of Preventive Medicine* 44, no. 1 (January 2013): 23–29, doi:10.1016/j.amepre.2012.09.056.

Index

About the Author

Jenna Wolfe served as the *Today* show's first Lifestyle and Fitness Correspondent and NBC News National Correspondent. Wolfe spent twelve years as a sportscaster before joining the *Today* show in 2007.

Her background, like her personality, is spirited. Born in Kingston, Jamaica, and raised in Port-au-Prince, Haiti, she moved to the United States in 1989, so her American pop culture references only date as far back as Duran Duran, *When Harry Met Sally*, and Michael J. Fox (all big that year). She is fluent in French and Creole and can ask you where the library is in Spanish (which, by the way, has never come in handy).

A self-proclaimed daredevil and thrill seeker, Wolfe is also a certified personal trainer, both on TV and in her spare time. Among her honors and accomplishments, she's most proud of receiving the distinguished IDEA Jack LaLanne Award (given to her in 2015 by the IDEA Health and Fitness Association, the world's leading organization of fitness and wellness professionals) for her contribution to the world of fitness, as well as the "Most Athletic Mom" award (given to her by her daughters).

Of all the adventures she's embarked on, motherhood is by far her favorite. She gave birth to Harper Estelle in 2013 and Quinn Lily in 2015. Jenna and her partner, Stephanie Gosk, have been beaming (and sleep-deprived) ever since.